The Nurse as Caregiver

for the Terminal Patient and His Family

The Nurse as Caregiver

for the Terminal Patient and His Family

EDITED BY

ANN M. EARLE, NINA T. ARGONDIZZO,

AND AUSTIN H. KUTSCHER

WITH THE EDITORIAL ASSISTANCE OF LILLIAN G. KUTSCHER

Columbia University Press   1976   New York

CHAPTER 17 originally appeared in Peter Koestenbaum,
Managing Anxiety: The Power of Knowing Who You Are,
© 1974, pp. 173–78. Reprinted by permission of
Prentice-Hall, Inc. Englewood Cliffs, New Jersey.

Library of Congress Cataloging in Publication Data
Main entry under title:
The Nurse as caregiver for the terminal patient
    and his family.

    Includes bibliographies and index.
        1. Nursing—Psychological aspects.   2. Terminal
care.   3. Death—Psychological aspects.
I. Earle, Ann M.   II. Argondizzo, Nina T.
III. Kutscher, Austin H.
RT86.N85   610.73'6   76-14441
ISBN 0-231-04020-2

Columbia University Press
New York   Guildford, Surrey
Copyright © 1976 by Columbia University Press
All Rights Reserved
Printed in the United States of America

❈ACKNOWLEDGMENT❈

The editors wish to acknowledge the support and encouragement of the Foundation of Thanatology in the preparation of this volume. All royalties from the sale of this book are assigned to the Foundation of Thanatology, a tax exempt, not for profit, public research and educational foundation.

Thanatology, a new subspecialty of medicine, is involved in scientific and humanistic inquiries and the application of the knowledge derived therefrom to the subjects of the psychological aspects of dying; reactions to loss, death, and grief; and recovery from bereavement.

The Foundation of Thanatology is dedicated to advancing the cause of enlightened health care for the terminally ill patient and his family. The Foundation's orientation is a positive one based on the philosophy of fostering a more mature acceptance and understanding of death and the problems of grief and the more effective and humane management and treatment of the dying patient and his bereaved family members.

DEDICATION

This book is dedicated with respect and admiration to all those in the profession of nursing.

The Foundation of Thanatology

CONTENTS

The Nurse as Caregiver

for the Terminal Patient and His Family

So live, that when thy summons comes to join
The innumerable caravan, which moves
To that mysterious realm, where each shall take
His chamber in the silent halls of death,
Thou go not, like the quarry-slave at night,
Scourged to his dungeon, but, sustained and soothed
By an unfaltering trust, approach thy grave,
Like one who wraps the drapery of his couch
About him, and lies down to pleasant dreams.

WILLIAM CULLEN BRYANT, Thanatopsis (1811)

Nursing and the Therapeutic Relationship

EILEEN M. JACOBI

When the dying were encouraged to face death in a "sustained and soothed" manner, the average life expectancy was less than 40 years. Ironically, in this final quarter of the twentieth century when the average life expectancy is 70, man is inclined to fear and deny the reality of death. Two million Americans die each year, and the care they receive is influenced by our society's less-than-healthy attitudes toward death. It has even been suggested that the "estimated social value" of the dying patient is a factor in the quality of medical and nursing care rendered. If characteristics such as age, intelligence, occupation, family position, and beauty determine an individual's social value and are equated with his potential to "serve mankind," the person ranking highest would receive the most attention and heroic efforts when his life was in jeopardy. Those graded in descending order on such a scale could expect a decreasing quality of medical and nursing care (Shusterman, 1973, p. 468). Browning and Lewis (1972) suggest that our youth-oriented society with its cure-directed system of health care militates against the adequate care of the dying.

Avoidance of patients is made possible by what Glaser, Strauss, and Quint (in Shusterman, p. 468) refer to as "nonaccountability" of terminal care. The significant implication of this absence of accountability is that medical staff are not legally bound to treat the dying patient in a psychological manner. Yet dying is a psychological as well as a biological process. Although the institution accepts responsibility for the biological care of the dying patient, it has not accommodated itself to his psychological needs.

Inasmuch as the primary focus of nursing care should be centered on patients, rather than on treatment of disease, nurses are the health workers who should help dying patients cope with contemporary fears of dying, preparing them to face death "sustained and soothed." Because of their accessibility to families, moreover, nurses are in a position to offer preventive, supportive, and therapeutic intervention during periods of family grief.

Therapy for a dying patient, whether or not he is totally aware of the seriousness of his situation, can help alleviate various anxieties and guilt as he faces death. Therapeutic intervention is not a tool to be used solely by the psychiatric nurse in his/her dealings with patients suffering from mental disorders. Indeed, all registered nurses are able to observe and distinguish a broad range of physical and socio-psychological problems. The nurse's help can frequently begin with a response to a concrete physical complaint and then evolve to investigating and interacting with the less tangible, emotional concomitants.

Today some form of nursing therapy is an inherent part of all nursing practice. To function effectively in a therapeutic role with the dying patient, a nurse must examine his/her attitude toward death, understand basic reactions to and stages of the dying process, and become skilled in verbal and non-verbal communication and listening. According to Travelbee (1971):

Nursing is an INTERPERSONAL PROCESS whereby the professional nurse practitioner assists an individual, family, or community to prevent or cope with the experience of illness and suffering and, if necessary, to find meaning in these experiences.

NURSE'S REACTION TO DEATH

A person's imminent death creates conflicts and tensions in those caring for him. The nurse's individual reactions to death inevitably affect his/her ability to give optimum care to a dying patient and his family. Exploring these reactions is essential to the nurse's professional growth and development.

Many hospital-based nurses who feel ill prepared to cope with the problems of the dying patient have suggested that schools of nursing provide insufficient training. Mervyn (1971) has stated that the lack of supportive emotional care for dying patients can be attributed to the nature of nursing education: "In helping students learn how to care for dying patients, nursing education has far to go. Students can list the physical care needed by a dying patient in detail, but are uncomfortable about any discussion of their own feelings about death."

Glaser and Strauss (1968) have made several recommendations for providing the nursing student with more opportunities to deal with personal reactions to death. These include broadening the scope and depth of terminal-care training in schools of medicine and nursing; explicit planning and review of the psychological, social, and organizational aspects of terminal care; and the encouragement of open discussion, among medical and nursing personnel, of the issues that transcend professional responsibilities for terminal care.

NURSE'S KNOWLEDGE OF DYING

Once the nurse works through personal feelings about death, recognizing the reactions likely to be touched off by an encounter with death, he/she must become sensitive to the stages of dying and aware of patterns of coping with death.

A patient's background, his health (both mental and physical), and his religio-philosophical orientation shape his attitudes toward death and dying. Responses to recognition and acknowledgment of impending death follow a continuum between psychological denial of death as a personal, natural, and individual occurrence and frank acknowledgment of death's certainty and imminence.

Glaser and Strauss (1968 pp. 41, 47) observe that the course of dying ("the dying trajectory") has various shapes and durations. They suggest that understanding the customary dying trajectories, as these relate to each nursing service, planning explicitly to cope with the various stages of the dying process, and examining the possible effect on staff would improve the nursing care rendered to every dying patient.

Kubler-Ross (1969) identifies five stages that the dying person experiences before his actual death: (1) denial and isolation (refusal to accept the terminal illness), (2) anger (Why me?), (3) bargaining (attempt to buy time with good acts), (4) depression (a reactive depression stemming from nonacceptance and/or a preparatory depression that comes from a grieving for future losses), and (5) acceptance (during a long dying period). A knowledge of what to expect as the individual reaches each stage enables the nurse to accept with more understanding the behavior common to dying patients. Moreover, Kubler-Ross points out that family members undergo similar stages of adjustment.

Nursing therapy is usually designated as direct patient–family care, for what influences one person also affects those with whom his life is intertwined. Since family reactions contribute much to the patient's response to his illness, the terminally ill patient cannot be helped in a meaningful way if his family, the primary group in his life, is not included.

A family may be prepared for the forthcoming death, persuaded to delegate responsibility for the dying individual to the hospital, coached in the proper modes of behavior while in the hospital, and helped in their grieving (Glaser and Strauss 1968, p. 151). In dealing with the family, it is important that the nurse have a clear understanding of the processes and patterns of grief.

NURSE'S RELATIONSHIP WITH DYING PATIENT

A nurse's ability to provide high-quality care for a dying patient is greatly enhanced by his/her ability to cope with personal feelings and to apply knowledge about the dying process. However, the patient may be most greatly comforted by the nurse–patient relationship. Feder (1965, p. 614) reports the greatest preoccupation of dying patients is not death, but rather the danger of progressive isolation and the development of a sense of aloneness. It is a fact that, the more our lives become surrounded by the unfamiliar and uncaring, the more we need authentic communication with a few people of significance in our lives (Bormann and Bormann, 1972, p. 15). It is therefore imperative that the nurse recognize the therapeutic benefits of simply establishing sound lines of communications with the dying patient and be alert to the cues by which terminal patients communicate their desire to explore death and dying.

Aronson (1959) states that care of the terminal patient should enable him to continue as a human being and maintain his role and identity and should keep him from becoming depressed. The ability to communicate is a basic requirement in any attempt at self-identity and fulfillment. Inasmuch as 70 percent of our daytime hours are normally spent communicating, it is important that dying patients be encouraged to seek out forms of communication.

The responsibilities of the nurse in "therapeutic" communications are twofold: (1) learning to recognize the needs of the patient who wants to talk about impending death and (2) developing a trusting relationship with the patient.

Many nurses rate talking with a dying patient as one of their most difficult tasks. Unfortunately, they assume that the desire to talk about death and dying reflects a need to fantasize what death is going to be like. In reality, the patient is seeking an individual with whom he can share his anxieties about the period of life that remains. If the nurse can establish a trusting relationship with the patient, even unpleasant things can be discussed openly, not without discomfort, but with a feeling of mutual satisfaction (Bormann and Bormann, p. 117).

Inasmuch as the role of the nurse combines speaker with listener, several things must be considered:

Communication is both verbal and nonverbal. Messages are conveyed verbally, vocally, and visually.

As a *speaker,* one of the most important ways to communicate nonverbally with a listener is by means of facial expression. Moreover, whether or not the speaker looks at the listener affects how the listener interprets what is said.

To listen is to do more than to hear. Listening is a mental function that involves perceiving a message.

Since speaking is elliptical, the *listener* must fill in gaps with personal understanding and experience. Interpreting body language, vocal symbols, and other relevant symbols is a listener's responsibility. Listeners often read into messages the meaning that fits their personal biases and interests.

Communication problems come about simply because people avoid talking about what really bothers them.

If a nurse is to assume a therapeutic role in caring for the dying patient, he/she must rely on the practical cues gained from an examination of personal reactions to death, a study of dying and grieving, and actual communication with the patient.

REFERENCES

Aronson, G. J. 1959. "Treatment of the Dying Person." In *The Meaning of Death,* ed. H. Feifel, pp. 251–58. New York: McGraw-Hill.

Bormann, E. G. and N. C. Bormann. 1972. *Speech Communication: An Interpersonal Approach.* New York: Harper & Row.

Browning, M. H. and E. P. Lewis. 1972. *The Dying Patient: A Nursing Perspective,* p. 62. New York: American Journal of Nursing Company.

Feder, S. 1965. "Attitudes of Patients With Advanced Malignancy." In *Death and Dying: Attitudes of Patient and Doctor,* pp. 614–622. New York: Group for Advancement of Psychiatry.

Glaser, B. G. and A. L. Strauss. 1968. *Time for Dying,* pp. 253–59. Chicago: Aldine.

Kubler-Ross, E. 1969. *On Death and Dying,* pp. 34–121. New York: Macmillan.

Mervyn, F. 1971. "The Plight of Dying Patients in Hospitals." *American Journal of Nursing* (October): 1988–90.

Shusterman, L. R. 1973. "Death and Dying: A Critical Review of Literature." *Nursing Outlook* 21 (July).

Travelbee, J. 1971. *Interpersonal Aspects of Nursing,* p. 4. Philadelphia: F. A. Davis Company.

1

Overview: Care, Cure, and the Challenge of Choice

JEANNE QUINT BENOLIEL

Quality of survival implies to me that the meaning of human existence is measured not by duration of life, but by the opportunities available to each individual to use to full advantage the special capacities designated as uniquely human. In the United States, the present system of health care (more properly, perhaps, a system of sickness care) places a heavy emphasis on duration of life, primarily because the goal of recovery carries top priority in the system.

In a profound sense, society today has created a cultural system for depersonalizing, specializing, and fragmenting human death and dying. From a sociological perspective, as Blauner (1966) has noted, this death system protects society from the disruptive impact of death by segregating the dying from the living and by developing bureaucratic procedures for managing death and dying as routine social matters. From a psychological and personal perspective, however, individuals who find themselves involved with death—whether as the person facing death, as members of the family, or as caregivers—are not provided with simple answers for the problems they encounter or with emotional support when the going gets tough. Rather, they find themselves ill prepared for the difficult problems and choices they meet. They find themselves caught in a complex social system that attaches high value to lifesaving procedures and technical activities and is poorly organized to offer personalized services to those who are dying.

The term quality of survival implies a shift in priorities away from an emphasis on recovery for recovery's sake toward an emphasis on person-centered goals. Achievement of the latter implies that care rather than cure is given primary status in the delivery of health care. This article examines the issues of care and cure as they pertain to the work of nursing. The discussion is organized into four general topics: differentiation of care and cure; special problems associated with death-related clinical situations; establishment of priorities in nursing services; and education of practitioners for human-centered practice.

CONCEPTS OF CARE AND CURE

To move toward converting care concepts into practical guidelines, I offer the following analysis of cure and care. Cure centers on the diagnosis and treatment of disease. In contrast, care is concerned with the welfare and well-being of the person. Cure deals with the objective aspects of the case, whereas care is concerned with the subjective meaning of the disease experience and the effects of treatment on the person. Cure has many origins in science and instrumentation and "doing to" people. Care has its roots in human compassion, respect for the needs of the vulnerable, and "doing with" people.

As a result of my work with patients facing death, I define personalized care as having at least three components. First, each patient has continuity of contact with at least one person who cares for him as a human being. Second, the individual is provided with opportunity to know what is happening and to participate in decisions affecting how he will live and how he will die. Third, the recipient of services has confidence and trust in those providing his care (Benoliel, 1972).

All health-care practitioners must find a balance between

the cure goal and the care goal. Changes in medical technology have brought new procedures and unusual techniques of treatment; hence, the options open to medical and nursing practitioners have increased in complexity. According to Potter (1973, p. 40), "the ethical problem is that of deciding when to intervene in the life of another person and when not to do so." For life-prolonging equipment and techniques, he suggests an ethical approach that advocates use of these techniques only under two conditions:

1. the situation is assumed to have a good chance of being only temporary, and
2. the individual has a good chance of living out a substantial fraction of his projected life span as an individual after recovery (Potter 1973, p. 41).

Since neither of these conditions is met in the case of the dying patient, additional guidelines must be developed. My own bias requires that the patient himself be involved in choices and decisions about his illness, treatment, and the circumstances surrounding his final days of living.

SPECIAL PROBLEMS ASSOCIATED WITH DEATH

By virtue of the positions they hold within the health-care system, nurses are often key people in finding the proper balance between care and cure. But the extent to which nurses exert leadership in creating humanizing environments for patients facing death is far from clear. Much in the literature suggests that nurses in general cope with death-related clinical problems by avoidance and noninvolvement (Reynolds and Kalish, 1974).

Inadequate Preparation for Death Work

These patterns of behavior are readily understandable if one recognizes that most nurses have been inadequately prepared to deal constructively with death and dying as clinical problems. Education for work in nursing has emphasized lifesaving activities, maintenance of professional control, and the avoidance of failure (Quint, 1967). Only recently have efforts been made to counteract the "culture shock" of socialization into nursing with explicit measures to assist new students in coming to terms with the psychosocial impact of becoming nurses (Wise, 1974). Much of the research on attitudes toward death suggests that nurses' attitudes may not be much different from those carried by the population in general. Folta (1965) found that nurses were ambivalent in their reactions toward death—viewing it as controlled and predictable in the abstract but high in anxiety when the threat became personal. Comparing ill patients with healthy subjects, Feifel and Branscomb (1973) found three levels of response to fear of death in both groups: repudiation of fear at the conscious level, ambivalence at the fantasy level, and outright aversion to death at the unconscious level.

Inadequate preparation for dealing with death is only part of the reason that nurses experience difficulty in coping with death-related problems. The settings in which nurses practice have been altered under the influence of specialization in medical practice, and changes in science and technology have increased the stresses and strains of work in which death and dying are central issues.

Death and Technology

Although degenerative diseases are the primary causes of death today, one cannot discount the contribution of accidents to deaths and near-deaths in hospitals. In 1969 in the state of Washington (*Washington Vital Statistics Summary.* 1970), accidents were listed as the fourth-leading cause of death, with an increasing proportion of these being associated with traffic incidents. One product of modern technology—the automobile—is responsible for a growing number of clinical situations that demand emergency services and that require hospital personnel to deal with the psychosocial problems associated with DOAs (dead on arrival), with deaths soon after arrival, and with decisions about the continuation or discontinuation of life-sustaining resuscitatory measures.

Science and technology have contributed to hospital practices in a second important way—through the development of high-risk procedures and equipment capable of keeping the physical body alive almost indefinitely. New forms of surgery, antibiotics and chemotherapy, advances in parenteral medication and treatment, and life-assisting devices all make possible the prolongation of living—and the prolongation of dying. Useful as they may be, these new technologies have added to the complexity of medical decisions when the threat of death is present, as Glaser (1970) has described.

High-Stress Work

Medical and nursing personnel have always been caught between two somewhat conflicting goals of practice: to do everything possible to keep the patient alive, but to do nothing to prolong pain and suffering uselessly. In my judgment, the availability of life-prolonging machines, organ transplants, and other extreme treatments has contributed to the development of hospital environments in which the first goal (lifesaving) has taken precedence over the second (relief of suffering), so that care of the person has become secondary to prevention of death.

There is also evidence to suggest that the intensive care setting may have negative outcomes for nurses as well as patients. Two recent articles have described in some detail the situational and psychological stresses and strains experienced by nurses assigned to such settings (Hay and Oken, 1972; Vreeland and Ellis, 1969). Intensive care wards are work situations marked by these conditions: repetitive exposure to death and dying; daily contacts with mutilated and unsightly patients; formidable and demanding work loads; limited work space; intricate machinery; and communication problems involving physicians, staff, and families. My observations suggest that nurses who cannot tolerate continuous assignment to these settings feel caught between the task of "lifesaving at all costs" and a desire to provide the patient a humane and dignified death. Especially upsetting to many are decisions to prolong the patient's life when he obviously is not going to survive.

Lifton's description of the war in Vietnam (1972) as an "atrocity-producing situation," resulting from exposure to a dehumanizing and meaningless experience that left many young American veterans with a sense of absurd evil, has been most impressive. Since reading Lifton, I have pondered the psychological and social consequences for nurses of continued exposure to the situational pressures of the ICU, which, it seems to me, create an intense conflict-producing situation. Gentry, Foster, and Froehling (1972), comparing nurses working on three intensive care settings with nurses on three nonintensive wards, found the ICU nurses in general reported more depression, more hostility, and more anger than non-ICU nurses did. It is my contention that intensive care nursing creates dehumanizing circumstances for the staff in that they must deal constantly with four critical conditions of work: conflicting expectations and demands; frequency of life–death decisions and their aftermath; information overload; and patients with high dependency on them for both lifesaving activities and personalized care (Benoliel, 1975).

Nonaccountability of Psychosocial Care

In addition to the development of special-purpose high-risk work settings, specialization has also created a great increase in the numbers of different types of health-care workers. As a result, the organizational structure of hospitals and other health-care delivery systems has become extremely complex. A major barrier to patient-centered care arises from the inadequate and ineffective communication among the many workers involved.

Although there is much talk among health-care workers in hospitals about the concept of teamwork, the organization itself tends to be structured so that each group of specialists interacts strictly within itself instead of engaging in conversation with members of other groups also involved in patient services. Often communication between groups takes place by such formal means as written orders on patients' records, so that there is no opportunity for informal meetings at which problems can be discussed and misunderstandings can be clarified. With so many people involved, authority and responsibility are difficult to pinpoint, and this deficit in accountability is most clearly apparent in the provision of psychosocial care to patients and families.

Lack of education in death and dying for all personnel, combined with the complexity of social structure, leads to a fragmentation of disciplinary responsibility for dying patients. In essence, the psychosocial care of people who find themselves in life-threatening situations tends to get lost in the shuffle. We need to recognize that the staff are held accountable for the goals that carry priority in the system—namely, the lifesaving goals of practice.

Inadequate understanding of the complex problem of giving personalized care contributes to the difficulty of establishing a system of accountability for the psychosocial component of patient care. There is a deficiency in education that, I believe, plays a tremendous part in maintaining this state of affairs. None of the health-care disciplines provides education and practice in the pragmatics of teamwork. Yet much of the work in health care today depends on the ability to function productively in a team relationship with other disciplines. Teamwork is especially critical in psychosocial care, where the "expert" needed by the patient or family may or may not be a physician. Teamwork, however, must be recognized as a necessary commodity by all members of the team if the goal of personalized care is to be achieved. Furthermore, practice at teamwork must be built into the educational system if health-care workers are to learn the what, when, where, why, and how of functioning in a coordinated, cooperative, and respectful way.

As I have tried to suggest, the problems associated with

death have increased in complexity. Reflecting the primary values of society, the health-care system places a high priority on the delivery of life-prolonging services. It has not been effectively organized to protect dying patients from social isolation or to assist them in achieving a dignified death. Rather, the present system of services perpetuates the general societal pattern of denying the reality of forthcoming death and leads to a depersonalization of experience for many during the final period of living. Let me comment briefly on two manifestations of depersonalized practices.

Depersonalization of Experience for Consumers

Whenever the family and/or the physician decide that a patient is not to be told the true state of affairs about his illness and future, a dilemma in communication is created for other health-care personnel and for the patient. For the staff, daily interacting with him, the problem of what to say appears whenever the patient tries to find out what is happening. The patient is denied the opportunity to participate in decisions about his own forthcoming death and to bring his life to a close in his own way.

Savard (1970) has pointed to the need for all paramedical workers to have a set of principles and guidelines governing their ethical and moral responsibilities to patients who are subjects in clinical and experimental research. I suggest that the need for such a set of principles in the case of the dying patient seems equally acute.

The assumption that the patient's right to be informed about the seriousness of his condition is the sole responsibility of the physician should, perhaps, be modified if the well-being of dying patients as human beings is to be protected. I do not intend, with this suggestion, to undermine the authority of the physician in diagnosing and treating disease. I do suggest that nurses and other health-care workers must be willing to accept responsibility for their choices and actions in the provision of terminal care if the human needs of the patient are to receive attention comparable to that currently given to lifesaving activity.

The reality that patient care in today's world is provided by groups of practitioners, who together provide services to patients, must be faced. It is clear that there are serious and difficult problems that confront medical and nursing practitioners when the threat of death is a critical and frequent feature of their work. The problem for health-care practitioners in general centers around the dilemma of how to reorder priorities in the ongoing daily services to people so that human concern and care do not get submerged under the prestige attached to lifesaving activity.

A second manifestation of depersonalized practice rests in the unrestrained use of medical technology to prolong life against the patient's wishes. As Kass (1971) has noted, the special expertise of the doctor with respect to the patients puts the doctor in a position of power to use the techniques of biomedical progress, often without informed consent. In order for the individual practitioner to set priorities, he must find a balance between the occupational goal of "performing a specialized service" for a client and the human goal of "sharing the final experience" with him. The practitioner's dilemma here is fundamentally ethical, and he should ask himself what each human being's rights and responsibilities are with respect to his own life and his own death.

ESTABLISHMENT OF PRIORITIES IN NURSING SERVICES

For all of us in the health-care disciplines, the fundamental ethical problem of practice is finding the balance between the care and cure goals. Potter (p. 41) has stated the problem in the following words.

The issue of intervention goes far beyond the matter of avoiding harm to the patient, or intervenee, in general terms. It involves the propriety of one individual or of society "managing" or intervening in the life of one individual or group of individuals, even with the best of intentions, and even when requested to do so by the individual or by society. The problem is to find the line that divides professional service, or friendship, or love in any of its forms from the many custodial relationships that destroy human dignity.

Making choices on the basis of morality rather than expediency is a necessary component of ethical practice. Indeed, the moral nature of health-care work requires that practitioners learn to differentiate between personal choices and professional choices in difficult care situations. Professional decisions that take account of the care needs as well as the cure needs of patients and families require knowledge of both the psychosocial and the physical consequences of the terminal disease. In cancer, for example, the need for care often extends over prolonged periods of time, and I want to use some special problems precipitated by cancer to focus attention on the personal needs of patients in the terminal stages of illness.

Special Problems Precipitated by Cancer

All of us in health care should be aware that cancer is a "dread" disease that carries fears of disintegration of the body and abandonment by other people. In fact, all of us carry these same fears, and we often encounter special problems in being open with cancer patients about what is happening to them and in letting them tell us about their concerns.

Cancer can be conceived as catastrophic in several ways, because it produces major changes in living for the individual and his family. For the patient, the diagnosis means learning to live with uncertainty. For the family, cancer can bring depletion of a family's monetary and psychological resources if living and dying continue for prolonged periods of time.

In formulating ideas about caring, nurses need to understand the special needs for assistance that come from the physical changes produced by or associated with cancer. One major difficulty for many comes from the fact that the treatment produces disfiguring outcomes or progressive physical changes that in turn affect the patients' functional capacities as social beings. A problem clearly associated with progressive cancer comes with physical deterioration of the body and the physical ministrations that must be performed by other people. The extreme emaciation associated with progressive disease can be difficult for the person to face in himself, and he is acutely sensitive to the fact that others have negative reactions to his appearance.

The inability to provide self-care in and of itself can be a humiliating experience, especially for someone who has been a proud and dignified person for much of his life. A particularly distasteful and awkward problem for patients comes with progressive loss of control of bladder and bowel. In essence, these changes can put the cancer patient back into infancy; psychologically and socially, the inability to control himself can be disastrously difficult for the adult ego to take. I am not sure that we who are caregivers appreciate just how difficult the experience must be to lose control over one's basic processes of elimination and to find oneself utterly dependent on others for help.

Another area of great concern for people with cancer has to do with any pain and discomfort triggered by the disease. Again, reliance on others is an important characteristic of the situation in which the cancer patient finds himself with respect to his pain. It has seemed to me that it is not just physical pain or the fear of pain that affects these people, although certainly these realities are often present. Perhaps it is also the fear of once again experiencing loneliness, compounded by the loneliness of facing death, an experience one must ultimately have alone.

A serious difficulty produced by progressive and metastatic malignancies comes with enforced dependency on other people, which reactivates all manner of unresolved problems in living and relating with other people. Persons who have great needs to be independent, for example, can easily react to the situation with hostility and frustration. Others may turn inward and withdraw in shame from interaction with those around them. Regardless of the pattern, enforced dependency is difficult for any adult who has spent much of his life being in a position of social control and dominance.

Another problem in the psychological domain comes from the tendency for families and health-care personnel to deny the cancer patient information related to his disease and his treatment. When information about diagnosis and treatment is withheld from a patient, his mind is free to conjure up all manner of fantasies. More important, he may sense that all is not well and he can develop a basic distrust of those providing his care. The patient must be kept informed if he is to participate actively in decisions affecting his continuing treatment, his stopping treatment, his hospitalization, and related matters.

A final problem associated with cancer stems from the requirement that one be institutionalized for the remainder of one's life. Many individuals would choose to die in their own homes if they were given the choice, and sometimes caregivers can help facilitate this goal. To do so means being able to negotiate effectively with both the patient and his family. Sometimes the needs of the patient and the needs of the family are not the same, and the nurse or physician must choose between the alternatives. Let me offer one illustration.

An elderly man dying of cancer at home was being seen there by a young physician. Both the old man and his family knew he had cancer, but by his choice, they engaged in the game of mutual pretense and did not talk openly about it. The old gentleman had willed the house to two of his daughters, who indicated they did not want to live there if he were to die at home. The physician suggested to them that they had better have their father taken to a hospital because he had no way of guaranteeing that the elderly gentleman would not die soon. This arrangement was satisfactory for the family, but the physician said he wanted to check with the elderly gentleman. When he mentioned the possibility of hospitalization, the old man said, "Oh, no—I want to die in my own home." The physician at this point made a decision to support the elderly gentleman's desire. He did then die in his own home.

Continuity of Care

Examination of the settings where cancer patients go for diagnosis and treatment shows that the nursing staff can play a central part in their lives. When patients are in institutions, the nursing staff often provide the main thread of continuity in human relationships and human contacts. It is they who are in a position to provide cancer patients with information and opportunities to share in decisions about day-to-day events. Whether in doctor's offices or clinics or on hospital wards, nurses can provide cancer patients with opportunities to talk about matters important to them. In particular, nurses and their associates have much to do with the provision of personal physical care and with ministrations to relieve pain and discomfort. The nursing staff provide physical assistance and personal contact that can make hospitalization an experience of personal comfort or deep despair.

The key position held by nurses having once been recognized, the next step means the establishment of priorities in nursing services. Acceptance of responsibility for continuity of care, for example, means the development of a system whereby access to necessary people and resources is continually available to patients. To implement the goal of care, the group must first define some standards for "measuring" the outcome. One set of guidelines can be taken from McNulty (1972), who has defined the needs of patients with advanced cancer in these words: "1) Relief from distressing symptoms, pain, and fear of pain. 2) An environment of caring where his demands can be met without his suffering the fear of being a burden. An environment where his individuality and integrity as a person can be maintained. 3) Time and opportunity to voice his fears, to come to terms with himself and his illness, to draw closer to his family."

Simple as these needs may sound, they are not simple to meet day by day; nurses who work where patients have advanced cancer know this. The problem centers around how to offer personalized services to more than one patient at a time, given the finite resources in people and money. The work of Cicely Saunders at St. Christopher's Hospice provides persuasive evidence that the creation of a caring environment for patients requires creation of a caring environment for the caregivers as well. One of the most vital characteristics of Dr. Saunders' work is the importance attached to the skills that every member of the staff brings to the enterprise.

To achieve the goal of continuity for each patient means that human needs for communication are recognized as sufficiently important to build and encourage human-to-human contact among staff and patients within the system. For this person-centered contact to take place, it seems clear that the staff members often require guidance in learning how to listen to patients and how to recognize the symbolic language they often use. Nurses who can allow cancer patients opportunities to become informed and participate in decisions about events in their lives must be knowledgeable about the patients' physical conditions, their responses to treatment, and their concerns about dependency on others. Most of all, however, nurses must place high value on the patients' right to know and to assist in decisions about their illness, their treatment, and their continuing life experiences.

The importance of psychological care cannot be overestimated. More than that, the interaction between psychological care and physical ministrations has perhaps not been given sufficient attention. Recognition should be given to the fact that valuable psychological care comes from being physically cared for in ways that ensure comfort. Much of a cancer patient's energy may be taken up with his physical responses, that is, nausea, vomiting, struggling for breath, and chronic pain, any one of which can be accentuated further by fear. Calm, confident, and unhurried assistance to patients experiencing these physical manifestations is one way a nurse can move toward achievement of the goal of care. There is perhaps no better way for cancer patients to experience con-

fidence and trust in their caregivers than in being provided
with relief from the miseries of their pain.

The Caregiving Process

Sometimes the most effective psychological care comes from
concerted attention to physical needs. The reality, of course,
is that people who happen to have cancer are faced with multiple physical, social, and psychological problems. More than
that, the problems they must solve vary according to whether
they are in the early stages of the disease, have been found to
have metastatic progression, or are in the terminal stages of
illness. The provision of care for the last group in particular
means that nurses as caregivers must be willing and able to
give a lot of themselves to situations that are not glamorous,
that at times may be distasteful, and that may often be
cogent reminders that fate may hold the same future in store
for them.

Saunders has shown that human care for people dying of
cancer can be provided when patients and caregivers alike
form a community of shared interests. I propose that the creation of caring environments on hospital wards, in extended
care facilities, and in nursing homes can come about only
when we in health care do more than give lip service to the
teamwork concept. We need to learn how to work together
effectively and how to respect the special contributions that
each staff member brings to the work. We need to move
away from a cure-oriented stance that emphasizes doing
things to patients, toward a care-oriented stance that respects
the consumer's right to share in decision making, that is *to do
with* patients.

Shifting health care settings toward the goal of care is not
a task to be taken lightly. In our society the cure goal and
cure activists carry top priority and influence all of our
health-care institutions. In contrast, the activities of care are
delegated to second place. In my judgment, it is no accident
that women and members of racial minorities are the primary
group engaged in direct patient care in nursing homes and

extended care facilities. Rather, the division of labor in health care effectively suggests that care services are less important than cure services and do not necessarily require special training or special expertise.

I would like to suggest the contrary. The provision of care services in the sense that I have been discussing them is a disciplined art that has its origins not solely in scientific knowledge but, perhaps more importantly, in humanitarian values and human ethics. The creation of caring environments requires that all members of the staff recognize that their contributions are valuable and essential to the goals and outcomes of the work to be done. The creation of caring environments depends on leadership that has at least two important attributes: flexibility of approach to problems and people, and a high sensitivity to personal and social events going on in the environment. Finally, there must be open recognition that the continual provision of care to dying patients can easily become routinized unless ways can be found for providing social and psychological support for the staff who carry the prime responsibility for direct care. The extent to which nurses can facilitate the development of caring environments in their work settings depends on their willingness to recognize that personalized care can come about only when the social system also provides personalized care for all members of the staff.

EDUCATION OF NURSING PRACTITIONERS

The art of nursing practice lies in finding an appropriate balance between the goals of care and cure. How does one educate students of nursing for the complex choices and problems that nurses face in their work with dying patients?

Knowledge Basic to Practice

There are several substantive areas to be emphasized if educational programs are to encourage the development of humanistically oriented nursing practices. To begin with, students need a broad base of knowledge about death as a human event with many dimensions—social, cultural, esthetic, emotional, psychological, and biological. In particular, they need to understand how historical and social forces over the past 100 years have shifted responsibility for managing dying from the family to the doctor and the hospital team (Aries, 1974). The opportunity to investigate death and dying as human experiences that have been described and portrayed in music, painting, poetry, and other art forms must be offered.

It is, perhaps, less important that they be exposed to detailed and specific facts than that they be exposed to a problem-solving and experiential approach in the use of scientific and other knowledge to better understand the many meanings of death in human experience. As they are introduced to various theoretical perspectives on death, dying, grief, and mourning, they can be encouraged to use their clinical observations for understanding the many ways by which people respond to death. As part of preparation for clinical practice, opportunities must be given students to identify their own reactions to death and dying and to share these feelings and reactions in a context of acceptance. As Wise (p. 43) has noted, students should know that it is acceptable to feel and express grief for the loss of a patient before they can move on to testing various nursing interactions with patients.

A central domain of knowledge is the introduction to general principles of sound clinical practice. In addition to learning the art of clinical observation, that is, physical and psychosocial assessments of states of wellness and illness, students should have a broad base of understanding of the social contexts in which nursing is practiced. They need exposure to situations that help them understand how cultural variations influence the behaviors of patients, families, and members of the health-care disciplines. They need to recognize that the implementation of care for dying patients often depends on how well nurses have learned to communicate effectively with physicians and with other members of the nursing staff. Perhaps most of all, students must have opportunities for developing the art of listening to patients under stress and for learning ways of providing psychological support that foster and encourage human dignity and human value.

Human-to-human communication and support lie at the heart of personalized nursing practice, but other activities are also important. Students need help in developing a set of principles to guide their selection of nursing interventions in practice. The curriculum should provide direction for students by identifying guidelines for translating the abtract concept of care into a concrete reality that makes sense in the real world of practice. Weisman's (1972) concept of *appropriate death* defined as "a death that someone might choose for himself—had he a choice" provides one starting point for developing a set of guidelines. Another comes from Koenig (1973), who believes that the key to practice is *preserving a viable quality of life,* which means helping the patient to have his own death on his own terms.

An area of knowledge central to learning the art of nursing practice deals with the influence of values and attitudes on human choice and human decision. If one accept's Potter's perspective that decisions about intervention are ethical problems and not solely clinical ones, then education for nursing practice must be concerned with helping practitioners of the future understand the moral implications of the choices they face. Especially important is the question of what to do when the goals of care and cure converge. In my opinion, students of nursing need help in understanding that personalized care of people facing death has its origin in an ethical stance toward the rights of individuals. The development of an ethical stance toward practice means that faculty and students have opportunities to recognize how much their own personal values and attitudes influence their choices and decisions in nursing practice.

Teaching–Learning Strategies

Education for ethical practice is fundamentally concerned with *making explicit* the problematic nature of the work that lies ahead. In my judgment (1968) the attitudes and behaviors of the faculty play a key part in the socialization through which students learn what nursing is all about and how they are supposed to behave. Clinical assignments should not protect students from involvement with the difficult problems that dying poses for nursing practice. Yet there should also be a backup support system that offers guidance for coping with difficult clinical problems and counseling services for assisting with the aftermath of traumatic encounters with death and dying.

If nurses of the future are to learn how to work constructively with physicians and other health-care personnel in finding a solution for death-related clinical problems, ways must be found to bring the various occupational groups together while they are still students. Krant (1974) believes that students from the different disciplines could profit from meeting for several hours of each academic week to share experiences and discuss major issues. In addition to maintaining dialogue about human caring, he sees these arrangements as offering opportunity for open deliberations about methods of making decisions and distributing power among the various groups engaged in providing care.

Of particular importance are educational experiences for both faculty and students that cause them to come to grips with the deep-seated influences of social values on institutionalized practices in health-care settings. Let me offer one example.

The management of pain is an extremely difficult clinical problem in the United States. We seem to be obsessed with what one might call the "fear of addiction" syndrome in our use of drugs for the management of pain. Among many people in health-care work, the standards of controlled use of pain medication are applied across the board, regardless of whether addiction does in fact make a difference. Nurses, in particular, seem to be caught up in a fear of giving the dose that puts the patient "over the edge" and brings about his death. My point here is that basic attitudes toward drugs and their uses, in combination with a high concern about personal negligence, interfere with the provision of effective pain control for many people with cancer. Education for nursing practice should make explicit the many difficult problems that nurses face when death is at issue, and thereby assist students in developing a problem-solving approach.

SUMMARY

As suggested at the beginning of this article, the term *quality of survival* implies a shift of priorities away from an emphasis on recovery for recovery's sake toward an emphasis on person-centered goals. Achievement of person-centered outcomes for dying patients and their families depends on practitioners who are committed to the preservation of human rights and human dignity in the face of many pressures toward dehumanization of patient care. It is my biased opinion that nurses occupy a singularly important position for influencing the dying patient's opportunity to have continuity of contact with at least one person who cares for him as a human being and his opportunity to know what is happening and to participate in decisions affecting how he will live and how he will die. Nurses can provide the kinds of direct care that cause the patient to experience confidence and trust in those providing his care. If nurses are to move in this direction, they must be willing to recognize the serious and difficult problems that face the dying patient and to accept the challenge of serving as advocate, helper, and friend toward the goal of dignified and personalized care for each patient on his own terms.

REFERENCES

Aries, P. 1974. *Western Attitudes toward Death*, pp. 85–107. Baltimore: Johns Hopkins University Press.

Benoliel, J. Q. 1972. "Nursing Care for the Terminal Patient: A Psychosocial Approach." In *Psychosocial Aspects of Terminal Care*, ed. B. Schoenberg et al., pp. 145–61. New York: Columbia University Press.

————. 1975. "Causes and Consequences of Dehumanization—A Commentary." In *Humanizing Health Care,* ed. J. Howard and A. Strauss, pp. 175–83. New York: John Wiley and Sons.

Blauner. R. 1966. "Death and Social Structure." *Psychiatry* 29 (November):378–94.

Feifel, H. and A. B. Branscomb. 1973. "Who's Afraid of Death?" *Journal of Abnormal Psychology* 81 (June):282–88.

Folta, J. R. 1965. "The Perception of Death." *Nursing Research* 14 (Summer):232–35.

Gentry, W. D., S. B. Foster, and S. Froehling. 1972. "Psychologic Response to Situational Stress in Intensive and Nonintensive Nursing." *Heart and Lung* (November–December):793–96.

Glaser, R. J. 1970. "Innovations and Heroic Acts in Prolonging Life." In *The Dying Patient,* ed. O. G. Brim et al., pp. 102–28. New York: Russell Sage Foundation.

Hay, D. and D. Oken. 1972. "The Psychological Stresses of Intensive Care Unit Nursing." *Psychosomatic Medicine* 34 (March–April):109–18.

Kass, L. R. 1971. "The New Biology: What Price Relieving Man's Estate?" *Science* 174 (November 19):779–88.

Koenig, R. 1973. "Dying vs. Well-Being." *Omega* 4 (Fall):181–94.

Krant, M. J. 1974. *Dying and Dignity: The Meaning and Control of a Personal Death,* pp. 130–54. Springfield, Illinois: Charles C. Thomas.

Lifton, R. J. 1972. "Home from the War—The Psychology of Survival." *The Atlantic Monthly* 230 (November):56–72.

McNulty, B. 1972. "Care of the Dying." *Nursing Times* (November 30).

Potter V. R. 1973. "The Ethics of Nature and Nurture." *Zygon* 8 (March):40.

Quint, J. C. 1967. *The Nurse and the Dying Patient.* New York: Macmillan.

————. 1968. "Preparing Nurses to Care for the Fatally Ill." *International Journal of Nursing Studies* 5:53–61.

Reynolds, D. K. and R. A. Kalish. 1974. "The Social Ecology of Dying: Observations of Wards for the Terminally Ill." *Hospital and Community Psychiatry* 25 (March):147–52.

Savard, R. J. 1970. "Serving Investigator, Patient and Community in Research Studies." *Annals of the New York Academy of Science* 169, no. 2 (January 21):429–34.

Vreeland, R. and G. Ellis. 1969. "Stresses on the Nurse in an Intensive Care Unit." *Journal of American Medical Association* 208 (April 14):332–34.

Washington Vital Statistics Summary, 2 1970, p. 48. Olympia, Washington: Department of Social and Health Services.

Weisman, A. D. 1972. *On Dying and Denying,* p. 41. New York: Behavioral Publications.

Wise, D. J. 1974. "Learning about Dying." *Nursing Outlook* 22 (January): 42–44.

Living, Dying, and Those Who Care

PART ONE

2

The Nurse as Crisis Intervener

SHIRLEY L. WILLIAMS

The last few years could be called the "Death Enlightenment" period as compared to the "Death Taboo" era of 10
years ago. The dominant themes of the mass of material ac-
cumulated in newspapers, magazines, and books and dissemi-
nated on radio and television and in seminars, college
courses, and so forth seem to be sadness, depression, and
pain. Yet a part of the milieu for the dying patient, his significant others, and the professional caregivers can also be
humor, lightness, renewed meaning, and an added sweetness
to life.

Whether death is at hand or only a phenomenon being
contemplated for some unknown future time, it is still a
unique experience for each individual. A young lawyer whose
specialty was assisting patients and hospitals with problems
associated with illness stated that, despite this professional
affiliation, he never really perceived the heights and depths of
a shortened lifespan until he himself experienced it.

When I approach the patient with an attitude that indicates, "I know about death and dying; here are the stages you
will be going through or should go through" and with an
array of advice, I fail to create a climate wherein the person
can be helped to resolve his difficulties with dying. If my attitude is, "Help me to understand and to empathize with you
in this unique experience of yours," the patient defines the

suffering and is provided with the needed catharsis. I, the listener, am better able to help him clarify solutions while gaining for myself new insights in human experiencing.

Within the clinical setting, nurses, more than any other health-care workers, are observers of human behavior and crisis interveners, from the first news that a patient's illness is terminal until his last breath. Yet often the nurse is the last to be consulted and the least recognized in the health-care and lay literature. Unfortunately, many nurses are too busy to analyze, categorize, and publish the extensive data on human behavior they have acquired. Although my experience is by no means so extensive as that of others, my observations and interventions are based on hundreds of nursing interviews and countless observations of the dying patient, his significant others, and the milieu of the hospital ward setting. Throughout 10 years of nursing practice, my major focus has been on the person critically ill from a variety of diseases, from trauma to cancer. More recently, my practice has been limited to a chemotherapy Cancer Research Ward where the emphasis is on the multidisciplinary approach for total patient care.

The nurse plays a major role in three crisis areas: where the patient experiences the crisis of a limiting and limited existence; where the family and significant others experience the crisis of impending loss; and where the attitudes and attributes of the nurse and other health-care workers confront the facts in the milieu of the dying patient. These are areas where assessments can be made and where personalized nursing can take place. Although the results of nursing interventions are not always the same or always subject to sophisticated statistical treatment, they can be evaluated in terms of observable patient behavior.

THE CRISIS OF A LIMITING AND LIMITED EXISTENCE

No amount of literature can prepare a person easily for an illness that portends diminished physical strength, altered physiological states, and obstruction of some or all of one's meaningful goals in life. Despite our recognition of death as a biological fact that must be faced, most of us confront the knowledge of its imminence with a fairly predictable state of shock. Because of the recent emphasis on being honest with the dying patient, once a person begins regularly seeking help for an illness, he is somewhat informed. Most health-care workers concur that dying patients have an inner aware-ness of an awesome process within them that needs verbal release (Brim et al., 1970; Kubler-Ross, 1969).

The anxiety of "knowing too much" that has been de-scribed by patients and critics of the recent honesty policy results, I feel, because inadequate support is given for the res-olution of problems and not because the patient should not have been told about his condition. A young patient once remarked to me, "I don't need so much help with dying but rather help with living until I die." Meinert (1968) has like-wise proposed that the focus of nursing should be on the liv-ing to be done.

Much of the suffering, anguish, and even pain—irrespec-tive of pathology—seems to be this task of "living until death." I suggest that much suffering could be reduced, if, instead of rushing to narcotics, sedatives, and funeral ar-rangements, we began to explore and define the suffering. Rather than the open statement of "needs to verbalize" on the Kardex, verbalization should be qualified. The proposal that nursing interventions can make a significant difference in pa-tients' pain experience is not new and has been more exten-sively researched by Diers et al.

For my interviews, I have learned that patients' problems can be categorized into 10 areas that, although they may not be comprehensive, can serve as assessment guides to aid the patient with his catharsis and guide the nurse to facilitate supporting, comforting interventions within the patient's own value system.

1. Complete and current information on bodily condition and proposed treatment modalities.
2. Restoration of hope.

3. Restoration and/or maintenance of meaningful interpersonal relationships.
4. Acceptance and readjustment to changes in body image, body comfort.
5. Restoration and reinforcement of basic life philosophy.
6. Resolution of financial crisis.
7. Recognition of creativeness and encouragement of continuing creativity.
8. Restoration and nurture of sense of humor, pleasurable activities.
9. Readjustment and/or transfer of major responsibilities and goals.
10. Resolution of dependence—independence conflict within realistic limitations of the illness.

1. *Complete and Current Information on Bodily Condition and Proposed Treatment*

Our age is not only one of enlightenment in regard to death and dying, it is also the age of the enlightened health-care consumer, and he is demanding more of a voice in decision-making about his own care. Patients no longer tolerate the anxiety created by the unknown. Most of the questions and concerns of the cancer patient are centered around "What is happening to me?" To tell a patient we will be "treating your disease with a medicine" is akin to telling him nothing and in actual violation of any reasonable informed consent. He wants to know where the tumor is on the X-ray, the name of the cell type, the relationship of the pain in the leg to the tumor in the chest, and so forth. In addition to factual information, patients appreciate knowing what sensations—for example, nausea, fatigue, pain—are usual and to be expected. Almost every patient understands individual differences and realizes that we cannot predict exactly how he will react, but he still appreciates some clues. When anxiety is great, it is the more difficult for him to remember details, and he asks the same questions over and over. As anxiety decreases, he is more capable of learning. If the nurse or doctor at this stage exhibits impatience, more anxiety is created within the patient, and his eventual cooperation is blocked. Patients who are continuously informed about their disease and treatment can use that knowledge to take better care of themselves. Some patients become as well or better informed than the health-care workers, and their challenges to and bargains with the team are a therapeutic game to them. Stewart Alsop, in his "memoir" of his battle with leukemia (1973), repeatedly comments on "knowing too much." In my opinion, his journalistic inquisitiveness would not have permitted him to remain ignorant. He enjoyed the game he could play with the doctors. Rather than too much knowledge, a more significant factor in his anxiety seemed to be the lack of support from professionals or other patients other than his matter-of-fact physician. Throughout the book I missed any reference to significant therapeutic conversation with nurses, psychologists, or social workers. Nurses were referred to only as "cheery" and hardworking. He tended to isolate himself from any supporting conversations with other patients. They were referred to as the "sad little group sitting in front of the television" or the "Notoire moribund." In our multidisciplinary setting, most patients and families are encouraged to seek the support that clarification of their questions by nurses, doctors, social workers, and psychologists can give. Weekly group discussions are held to enable the patients and their families or friends to share coping strategies, knowledge, and support methodologies with a nurse, psychologist, and social worker, and with each other.

The patient who must experience both the good and the adverse effects of treatment, who must completely rearrange his life accordingly, seems the most logical person to have the most significant vote in direction of treatment and/or comfort measures. He should have the information that will enable him to make a proper decision for himself. The decision may not be consistent with what the health team thinks is best, but they do not live in his body nor will they support his survivors. A young father, exhausted by a life-threatening kidney disease and painful crippling osteoarthritis, decided against receiving any treatment for his metastatic lung cancer, and his wife and nine children concurred with his decision. His death was quick and peaceful rather than painful, expensive, and prolonged. Yet a chronic schizophrenic who was considered to be almost emotionally unfit for treatment found chemotherapy one of the more exciting challenges in his life (in addition to other cancer fads he could read about and fit into our regimen).

2. Restoration of Hope

Restoration of hope begins as soon as the patient is made a partner in his own care. Realistic hope is not hope for cure or life forever but hope to achieve short-term to moderate-length goals, pleasures, or other meaningful activities. Some acknowledge that they use the mental mechanism of "hope for a cure" or denial of the disease for periods of time, but they recognize these as mental "tricks," not the reality. To destroy hope or to insist that the patient not have these temporary intellectual devices is to damage very important coping mechanisms. Deprived of hope, patients begin a quick downhill course irrespective of physiological pathology (Frankl, 1959; Jourard, 1971). Hope and the will to live seem to depend also upon the attitudes and perceptions of what is happening by family, significant friends, and influential members of the health-care team (Eisman, 1971; Wallace, 1961). If everyone thinks the patient is too far gone, too belligerent, or in too much pain, then he, too, loses hope. Even if the patient has not lost hope, the withdrawal of love and touch or the pain of sensory and social deprivation significantly reduce any will to live. Unfortunately, people still tend to withdraw and separate themselves from the patient when the cause is hopeless. I have seen patients who, so long as someone treated them as still living, have maintained a will to live, a will to enjoy one more cigarette, one more kiss, one more new joke, or one more smile from a grandchild, until the cancer snuffed out every single cell. A relative of one patient stated to me that, as long as people thought the patient was in a coma, he remained silent and seemingly comatose, but he could still manage a smile and a squeeze of the hand for her. Tears came to his eyes when anyone mentioned that hope was gone. In reference to hope, Alsop states, "A man will die more easily if he is left a little spark of hope that he may not die after all" (1973, p. 74).

3. Restoration or Maintenance of Meaningful Interpersonal Relationships

Pain, disability, and an uncertain future do not make one the cheeriest of companions, and yet warm personal relations are sometimes more valuable than narcotics and tranquilizers in reducing pain and easing tension. Although any person's relationships enter a crisis period no matter what state they were in before the crisis, skillful counseling by the health-care team at strategic times during the patient's hospitalization can strengthen and even improve relationships. The goal is not to emphasize what has been wrong or to make major changes, but rather to encourage and promote positive attributes. I feel we need to do research into the elements of the strong, close, supportive relationships when we observe the marked increase in the longevity of the patient who is well cared for and the marked decrease of tension when the spouse, relative, or friend remains near.

Friendships on the ward among the patients are especially treasured and useful. Group discussion, group games, and creative projects to foster relationship increase morale and decrease loneliness. Although there is grieving and a sense of loss when a friend dies, the consensus is that the friendship has enriched all who have shared it. The health-care team needs to support these interpersonal relationships.

4. Acceptance and Readjustment to Changes in Body Image, Body Comfort

Although many illnesses imply a chronic, debilitating downhill course, none seem to possess the same contexts of grimness and hopelessness that cancer does. The word itself projects an image of a wasting, odoriferous, pain-wracked body, with a rejection of self and rejection by others. The amount of shock and self-rejection associated with body disfigurement depends on how the person defines himself in terms of his physical body in total or in part. In some, any mutilation of the body is unthinkable, in others a colostomy or mastectomy is acceptable, but a laryngectomy is a serious crisis. A 70-year-old female patient accepted a mastectomy with no problems, but the metastatic pathological fractures that limited her independent existence resulted in an unresolved mental anguish, not to mention severe pain.

The most significant step toward helping the patient accept changes in his body image is his acceptance of support from the nurse who manages his care after the first body change operation. Assisting the patient to a restoration of as much normality as possible and as soon as possible (such as an immediate breast prosthesis) helps reduce any rejection by herself and others and any "conditioning," that her body is a terrible problem. Because of unpredictable colostomies, tracheostomies, and fulminating lesions, the uniformed nurse, unafraid of getting her hands "dirty," is a comforting sight for the patient, despite what our psychologist and psychiatric nurse colleagues claim about the sterility and coldness of white uniforms.

A patient may need help with personal hygiene to help reduce social rejection. Odors should not be masked with other odors; instead, regular tub baths should be provided and decaying tissues should be irrigated. Palliative, diverting colostomies and ileostomies can also provide that patient with a cleaner, more manageable body. Colostomy clubs, "Reach to Recovery" for mastectomy patients, and other such organizations are invaluable as social supports.

The patient can be enlisted as a partner in devising ways he can remain comfortable and maintain the highest level of well-being possible (Dunn, 1972; Oelbaum, 1974). It may mean using an old familiar cough syrup (judged medically as ineffective) or advocating squatting for perineal pain or for easier breathing. Occasionally, the patient should be allowed to persuade his doctors to lengthen the days between treatments or to skip a treatment in exchange for a beneficial retreat to the woods. If the patient incurs rejection because of these behaviors, his suffering is only intensified. Copp (1974) found in her studies of patients in pain that, unfortunately, many nurses and health-care workers tended to reject these patient-initiated coping mechanisms as unacceptable or impractical.

Ultimately, if the patient's family or significant others can accept him and his ideas as much as possible, the patient can more easily and finally accept and maintain himself in some degree of comfort. Group sessions with patients and spouses can increase tolerance of bodily discomfort, odors, and odd ideas.

5. Restoration and Reinforcement of Basic Life Philosophy

Every individual has a life philosophy. Many people, however, are unable to verbalize their thoughts when first asked, but dying patients definitely begin to review their value system, codes of ethics, and religious beliefs during such a crisis situation. I have found much anxiety exists if the patient's ideal values conflict with the values as he has practiced them, or if he experiences social, cultural, or family rejection because of different beliefs.

It might seem that a clergyman, a psychiatrist, or a psychologist might be the more appropriate person to resolve whatever conflicts about value system the patient may have. However, I have found that patients are most open and least threatened by the nurse, particularly if she is secure with her own life philosophy and nonjudgmental in her attitude. She is also more readily available when the patient is first likely to verbalize his concerns, that is, during the long evening and night hours or when he is receiving nursing care.

The nurse must first help the patient focus on the values and codes he has been able to keep in line with his ideal, rather than on "things he ought not to have done." There is neither time nor ego strength for major personality reorganization (Koenig, 1974). If the multidisciplinary support is strong and nonjudgmental and the person is made to feel good about himself, he can sometimes make major changes in life style and interpersonal relations that can improve his psychological functioning and make him more comfortable. Collaboration among all disciplines is therefore a very important second step for resolving conflicts.

If the patient feels that his whole life has been a mess and it seems impossible to reconcile this area of conflict, interviews with family members, friends, and clergy might reveal more positive aspects of the person's life. I recall spending considerable time with one woman as she related what a miserable person she had been until she convinced me she had left not so much as a trace of goodness in her life's path. Interviews with her husband, clergyman, and neighbors revealed, however, that she had a rich legacy of kind deeds. The basic conflict was with her parents' lifelong nonacceptance of her marriage and childlessness; these overshadowed her feelings about her entire ethical behavior. Short conferences were held with her husband and a favorite niece summoned from a neighboring state. All their efforts were then directed toward reminiscing with her about happy times and her good deeds so that the positive aspects of 40 years of marriage and 60 years of life could be impressed upon her. Her restlessness, vomiting, and verbalization of discontent with herself did decrease as a result.

Although most people base their philosophy of life on a religious faith, I have encountered a number of true agnostics and atheists. I have yet to see with certainty that there is any difference in suffering, serenity, or acceptance of death between religious and nonreligious persons. In addition to a person's intrapersonal conflict with his philosophy, he can experience a degree of social rejection if his beliefs are incongruent with those of his family, friends, or culture. Atheists and agnostics experience rejection, especially when they are expected to "see the light" and do not. The goal is to help the person feel content or to reconcile him to the belief that gives him the most inner peace, not to convert him or admonish him about what he should believe (Kavanaugh, 1974).

On the other hand, most patients find comfort in talking about their religion, and one has to set aside admonitions such as "Never discuss religion or politics."

6. Resolution of Financial Crisis

Chronic illness usually precipitates a financial crisis, even when there is adequate insurance or hospital care in a government-subsidized hospital. Unless a family is able to work out a new financial system or receive assistance in resolving this crisis, all members undergo a traumatic experience. The nurse may or may not be the major counselor in this area, but she might be the first to assess finances as a problem area and direct the patient for proper advice.

7. Recognition of Creativity or Encouragement of Continuing Creativity

Complicated treatment regimens, frequent hospitalization, and ultimately pain, weakness, and shortness of breath inhibit or prevent patients from pursuing their normal activities. Their sense of worth tends to decline, and their physical and emotional suffering to increase unless creative activities can be introduced in a new focus. If the person has been previously too busy for creative activities, it is not too late to try out his talents. Praise, materials, and group process can bring out budding talent in even the most reluctant patients. In hospitals where there is a Department of Occupational Therapy, the nurse may assume a secondary role, but she still may become a supporting and enthusiastic admirer of the patient's creations.

The relatives of one patient, who lived for two years longer than expected, felt a large part of his will to live and cheerful disposition was due to his new hobby of carving animals in wood. He also left his family a beautiful visual legacy.

8. Restoration and Nurture of Sense of Humor, Pleasurable Activities

Cancer wards and any other chronic illness wards need not be humorless settings; although the terminally ill may not have much to be happy about, they can enjoy a good laugh and survive the tedious days better if their sense of humor is nurtured (Alsop 1973 p. 149). A sense of humor can emerge if the nurse and other health-care workers convey genuine warmth and allow for adequate ventilation of the sadness and anger that accompany the illness. Sometimes patients' humor takes a wry twist; for example, a group may joke about how they will look in the coffin. In our setting, our housekeeper is one of the prime teachers and activators for nonjudgmental warmth and humor.

Pleasurable activities, while strength permits, also reduce tedium and suffering. A young father of two who looks normal and healthy enough to be gainfully employed has stated he looks that way only because of the inner peace he finds fishing and working with other hobbies. When he was trying to fit gainful employment in between cancer chemotherapy treatments, which make him very ill, he was unhappy with himself and felt himself sinking physically. Because he has "tightened his belt" and reoriented his values, the family feels he will live longer and be a more useful father and husband, despite the American cultural belief that the male must work and support his family.

9. Readjustment or Transfer of Major Responsibilities and Goals

As long as a patient feels he can continue living as usual, he should be encouraged to do so. When shortness of breath, weakness, or prolonged treatment make living more difficult, he needs to educate others and transfer to them his major responsibilities at work and at home. This is a very difficult time for the patient and requires much "ego massaging" by his significant others. Physically disabled persons can still be the "brains" and let others be the hands and feet, although this is difficult for the farmer, construction worker, or busy mother. Some patients tend to reminisce endlessly about past physical feats, achievements, and responsibilities, but if this can be recognized as a useful coping mechanism for a difficult adjustment, tolerance and patience can come more easily. Encouragement of creative activities is also an important bridge at this time.

10. *Resolution of Dependence–Independence Conflict within the Limitations of the Illness*

A valued American trait is self-reliance and fear of dependence. It is an ideal by which we judge all of humanity. As a result, the dependency resulting from a serious illness nearly always precipitates a loss of self-esteem and loss of social respect. Resolution of this conflict depends upon how significant others and health-care workers emphasize independent skills and gracefully accept the patient's dependency. Hsu (1961) states that man must live in dependence in varying degrees in order to survive. Nonacceptance of dependency can lead to discomfort and a more rapid decline. No one should force dependency beyond what is absolutely necessary, but acceptance of help should be encouraged when it is obvious that the patient may expend all his energy in barely maintaining activities of daily living. I have seen patients die uncomfortable, lonely deaths because of their refusal to accept dependency. In contrast, patients who have accepted it without compromising what they can comfortably do for themselves experienced a more comfortable, extended life, and their significant others felt fulfillment.

It is important that the nurse be nonjudgmental; the motivation for this attitude is not to reform the patient but to help him put his affairs in order, decrease his anxiety and suffering, and live more fully until he dies. The process is not a question-and-answer interview, but rather several in-depth conversations. The openness and depth of information revealed by the patient seem to be controlled by the genuineness, openness, and warmth of the nurse. This observation is consistent with the observations of Jourard (pp. 179–188) on nurse–patient relationships.

THE CRISIS AS EXPERIENCED BY THE FAMILY

The dying patient cannot be considered out of the context of his family and/or significant others. His acceptance of his situation and his length of survival may depend on their ability to cope. Support of the family, too, is aimed at their positive actions, not their nonsupporting ones. The crisis can be a growth-promoting experience for the entire family.

Caine (1974) has emphasized the growth that can be achieved by the crisis if repeated open verbalization and sharing of the bereavement experience take place. (These insights, however, did not come to her when she felt she could have made the most effective use of them.) Certainly the nurse is in one of the most advantageous positions to facilitate verbalization. To promote openness, I never ask a spouse, friend, or relative to leave the room if I can possibly avoid it. I give explanations and counseling to the patient and his family at the same time.

Family group sessions seem particularly valuable in promoting openness among family members and between families with common problems. Either group can be helped by health-care workers, or patients and families can seek out a group like "Make Today Count," originated in Burlington, Iowa, by Orville Kelly, a cancer patient.

One can readily see the ambivalent love–hate conflict that exists in all relationships when working with families. If positive aspects of a person or a relationship are not encouraged at a crisis time, overwhelming hate and discontent can emerge to such a degree that these feelings can arouse severe suffering in the patient and guilt in the survivors. One can speculate, as my colleague Goudsmit (1960) has, that legalized euthanasia might effect a person's demise before he wished it or while he was still a useful, productive human being. He further states,

Life is too short as it is; companionship too rare and too fleeting, sympathy too scarce and too cheap, compassion too much a thing for the other fellow to practice; selfless devotion too much a mere topic for homiletic histrionics. . . . life is too precious . . . yes, too sacred to take it away from any one fellow human being for any reason or under any pretext whatsoever.

ATTITUDES AND ATTRIBUTES OF NURSES AND OTHER HEALTH-CARE WORKERS

The nurses and health-care workers who seem to have the least difficulty and the most job satisfaction in interacting with dying patients seem to have some or all of the following characteristics:

1. Comfort with their own philosophy of life, religion, or value system.
2. Comfort with their concept of their own body image and sexuality.
3. Sense of humor that is not buried too deep in their seriousness of purpose.
4. Ability to converse nonjudgmentally with patients who have a variety of value systems.
5. Ability to listen actively, encouraging expressive feelings of the patient.
6. Lack of overreactiveness to strong odors, malformed bodies; no restriction of "hands on" interventions to bodies so needful of touch.
7. Ability to diagnose sources of physical discomfort and anxiety and to propose interventions or solicit help from other disciplines.
8. Ability to bear with the coping mechanisms of patients or calmly sit out agitated or angry behavior.

The experience of having had a close friend or relative die or of having been stricken with a serious illness themselves in which they contemplated their own demise and subsequent changes they would make seems to help these characteristics evolve. They are reinforced as the nurses are rewarded by the gratefulness of patients and their families. Certainly, the nurses themselves can use support and warmth from their families, friends, colleagues, and supervisors to promote their self-actualization, which in turn can be used to assist the patient.

In addition, the nurse can promote multidisciplinary communication of the variety of value systems and opinions that can meld for the common cause. The practical humanists who encourage the patient and his family to "give up" need to be balanced by the romanticists who encourage a few more memories of touching and tenderness. Basic medical and nursing management as well as research regimens to prolong life may not be considered as inhumane or unromantic but seen rather as the patient's legacy to research until a cure or significant prolongation of life for others can be achieved.

No one remains the same as a result of working with dying patients and their families. Human growth and renewed sweetness to life are inescapable gifts for those who elect to give care and hope to these fellow beings.

REFERENCES

Alsop, S. 1973. *Stay of Execution.* New York: J. B. Lippincott.

Brim, O. G. et al., 1970. *The Dying Patient.* New York: Russell Sage Foundation.

Caine, L. 1974. *Widow.* New York: William Morrow and Company.

Copp, L. A. 1974. "The Spectrum of Suffering." *American Journal of Nursing* 74 (March):491–95.

Diers, D. et al. 1972. "The Effect of Nursing Interaction on Patients in Pain." *Nursing Research* 21, No. 5 (September–October):419–28.

Dunn, H. L. 1972. *High Level Wellness* (7th ed.). Arlington, Virginia: Beatty Ltd.

Eisman, R. 1971. "Why Did Joc Die?" *American Journal of Nursing* 71 (March):501–3.

Frankl, V. E. 1959. *From Death Camp to Existentialism.* Boston: Beacon Press.

Goudsmit, A. 1960. "Euthanasia Can Never Be Justified." Unpublished speech to Ohio Torch Club.

Hsu, F. K. 1961. "American Care Value and National Character." In *Psychological Anthropology,* pp. 209–29. Homewood, Illinois: The Dorsey Press.

Jourard, S. 1971. *The Transparent Self.* New York: Van Nostrand, Reinhold and Company.

Kavanaugh, R. 1974. "Facing Death." *Nursing* 74 (May):39.

Koenig, R. 1974. "Dying vs. Well-Being." *Nursing Digest,* no. 5 (May):52.

Kubler-Ross, E. 1969. *On Death and Dying.* New York: Macmillan.

Meinert, N. 1968. "The Cancer Patient: Living in the Here and Now." *Nursing Outlook* 16:64–69.

Oelbaum, C. 1974. "Hallmarks of Adult Wellness." *American Journal of Nursing* 74 (September):1623–25.

Wallace, A. 1961. "Mental Illness, Biology and Culture." In *Psychological Anthropology,* ed. F. Hsu, pp. 255–92. Homewood, Illinois: The Dorsey Press.

One sees clearly the strength and dignity of human beings, the deep altruism, the positive qualities that exist at all levels of personality. Working with people who are under the hammer of fate (death) greatly increases one's respect for them and makes one proud to be a human being.

(LeShan, 1969).

3

The Terminally Ill Child, His Parents, and the Nurse

LUCY WARREN

The study of the psychological and emotional aspects of terminal illness is relatively new in medicine, nursing, psychiatry, and sociology. Before the mid-1950s, most available literature on the dying person dealt with the physical aspects of care. "Emotional care" was left to the clergy, for until that time most patients with a diagnosed fatal disease were doomed to die. Because of current advances in medical research and practice, the lives of these patients can be extended for even many years. This interim between the diagnosis of a terminal illness and the patient's death was soon realized to be traumatic for the patient, his family, and all those who worked with them. It was almost as if, by the discovery of cures for one ailment (immediate death), the door was opened to another ailment: the physical and psychological symptoms of anticipated loss and grief.

Pediatric patients who used to die at a very young age with cystic fibrosis, blood dyscrasias, and other incurable diseases are now being kept alive for months or years, often with no sign of their illness apparent to the untrained observer. To the medical personnel, the family, and sometimes even the children, however, the ultimate and untimely death is a known prognosis, often difficult to face and to accept. Knowledge of the best ways to help families cope with a terminally ill child becomes as important to the professional as knowledge of the physiology of the disease. To provide an overview of this knowledge as it relates to the child and pediatrics, I focus on the terminally ill child; his awareness of and means of coping with his own illness; his family and their means of coping; and finally, the role of the nurse in the care of both the terminally ill child and his family. (The phrase *terminal illness* refers to any illness for which there is no known cure and from which the child will ultimately die.)

THE CHILD

No one knows exactly how a child perceives death. Although one author (Marlow, 1969) states as fact that "to a child in the preschool period the idea of death as a physical fact is beyond his level of understanding," this must be questioned. This statement represents only one viewpoint. An understanding of children's perceptions of death must be reached from the research and experiences of many investigators.

Infants and Toddlers (0–2½ years)

Normal, healthy infants and toddlers have no concept of death, according to Gesell and Anthony (in Kastenbaum, 1969, p. 94). Kastenbaum, however, discussed Adah Maurer's suggestion that an infant's experiences and behavior do help him to begin to relate to a state of nonbeing (1969, p. 95). In playing a game such as peek-a-boo (meaning "alive-or-dead" in Old English), and in going to sleep and waking up, the child experiences being and nonbeing, even though he cannot conceptualize the experiences as being analogous to death. Circumstances surrounding these "insignificant" childhood experiences help mold the child's later conceptions of death, and a sense of security is thought to be vital if the child is not to fear death or nonbeing in a neurotic way in later life.

Furman (1964) believes a two- or three-year-old child can understand death as a concept, if the mother can realistically discuss it with him as it involves the loss of life in objects he is not closely related to. Furman suggests that parents begin discussing death with their children at this young age, before a close relative, family member, or pet dies.

Whatever the young child's understanding of death as a concept, it is clear that separation from the mother can arouse profound anxieties in children, anxieties similar to those caused by death itself. Bowlby's work (1960) with the grief experienced by hospitalized two and one-half year olds describes three phases of grief: protest, despair, and denial or detachment. For the terminally ill child who is younger, this separation from the mother appears to cause more anxiety than the illness or the painful procedures often involved in treatment. Knudson and Natterson (1960b) report that terminally ill infants and toddlers seem to have a generalized anxiety that is decreased only when the mother is present. If the mother is not present, the child is reported to be irritable, withdrawn, and socially regressed, often having problems with sleeping and feeding.

Hence, it would seem that infants and toddlers are fearful and anxious when separated from their human source of security (mother, in most cases) and that the presence of a concept of death is unusual in this age group.

Preschoolers (2½–4 years)

Most writers agree that preschool children are more curious than concerned about death, for a child at this age seems to believe that death is reversible rather than a final event (Nagy, 1959). What the child does not understand or finds frightening, he can explain away by magic or fantasy. Hence, the pet or person who dies is only "living somewhere else." Kastenbaum (1969, p. 100) goes further and says that a child of this age also believes that death is accidental when it does occur, for the child cannot appreciate that it is inevitable for all living things, including himself.

But what if the preschooler is terminally ill? As with infants and toddlers, the preschooler's primary fear seems to be separation from his mother, for the concept of death is still somehow equated with separation in this age group (Knudson and Natterson, 1960a, p. 485).

Early School Age (5–9 years)

By the time a child is five years old, he has begun to see that death is a final, inevitable, universal, and personal event (Kastenbaum, 1969, p. 101). Nagy (1959, p. 95) reports that the child from five to nine sees death as a "person," an external thing. Nagy studied 378 well children living in Budapest in 1948:

Either they believe in the reality of the skeleton man, or individually create their own idea of a death-man . . . who is invisible to them. This means two things: (a) it is invisible in itself, as it is a being without a body; (b) we do not see him because he goes about in secret, mostly at night.

Both Nagy and Kastenbaum postulate that at this age the child cannot quite cope with the fact that death is inevitable for himself, even though he knows this as a fact, and so the child creates a means of escape (Nagy, pp. 95, 96):

The child already accepts the existence of death, its definiteness. On the other hand, he has such an aversion to the thought of death that he casts it away. From a process which takes place in us, death grows to a reality outside us. It exists but is remote from us. As it is remote, our death is not inevitable. Only those die whom the death-man catches and carries off. Whoever can get away does not die.

When the child from five to nine has a terminal illness, he must put aside his beliefs that death is an external, escapable thing. A study by Waechter (1971) found that all 16 children (between six and ten) hospitalized with a terminal illness showed high levels of generalized anxiety, though only 2 of them knew their diagnosis. In the control group of non-terminally ill hospitalized children, only 50 percent showed high levels of anxiety. Another study (Binger et al., 1969) found that terminally ill children over the age of four presented evidence to their parents that they were aware of the seriousness of their disease, their fears of separation, pain, and disfigurement were great. Knudson and Natterson (1960a, p. 485) found terminally ill children in this age group less fearful of separation and most fearful of pain and disfigurement.

Thus we see the child of early school age is still struggling to come to terms with the concept of death, usually preferring to ignore it and concentrate his energy on mastering the realities of daily life. If he must think about death, he still prefers to think of it as something from which he can escape; but if death becomes a reality to him in the form of his own terminal illness, he becomes very frightened and anxious, focusing his concerns more on his own body (i.e., fear of mutilation) and its comfort and safety than on a fear of death.

Late School Age (9 Years to Beginning of Adolescence)

By this age, normal children have definite concepts of time, space, quantity, and causality. They can differentiate between the animate and the inanimate, and their egocentricity has decreased. Death as a concept can now be expressed in words that show their understanding of death as the final and inevitable outcome of life. One nine-year-old child, when asked how children would feel if a loved one died, replied:

They would cry and cry. They would cry for a month and not forget it. They would cry every night and dream about it, and the tears would roll down from their eyes and they wouldn't even know it. And they would be thinking about it and tears just running down their eyes at night while they sleep (Fishman, 1968).

The authors previously mentioned agree that the nine-year-old child is capable of having the same concepts of death as the adult. Consequently, it is with this age group that the serious question arises of whether or not the terminally ill child should be told his diagnosis. Because a child of this age still *looks* like a child, it is hard for most professionals and families to believe that his concept of death is similar to an adult's and that he should, therefore, be treated like an adult in this regard.

Studies based on impressions adults have about terminally ill children of this age have indicated that only 30 percent of these children showed anxiety and that the children reacted with an air of "passive acceptance and resignation," rarely showing an overt concern about death (Morrisey, 1965; Richmond and Waisman, 1955). However, when the children themselves are observed, the results are strikingly different. Karon and Vernick (1965), studying 51 terminally ill children at the National Cancer Institute, found that open discussion of the truth with support for the child, the family, and the staff was the best policy for children over nine years of age. When these children were not told the truth, severe behavior problems resulted. Knudson and Natterson (1960a, p. 485), report findings similar to those of Karon and Vernick.

It would seem that the older school-age child is ready to deal with death, even his own, in terms of his "adult concept of death." But the child's need for support from a trusted adult, preferably a parent capable of dealing with his own feelings about the death of the child, cannot be overemphasized. Any dying person needs open support, encouragement, and love; this is especially true for the nine-year-old "adult-like child."

Adolescents

Adolescents are young adults in terms of a concept of death, perceiving death with the same understandings, fears, and concerns of any adult. Most healthy adolescents appear too busy to think about death, but just as adults worry about death, or even at times desire it, so do adolescents. Kastenbaum (1959) points out, however, that while the adolescent is capable of considering death in adult terms and may think about it, he tends to consider death as a remote possibility for himself. At a time when living is so intense and the "now" is so important, any threat to his life is likely to engender a great deal of rage in the adolescent. Unable to deal with this rage and preoccupied with the "now," the terminally ill adolescent tends to focus on his symptoms and often worries more about whether his hair will fall out from the medications than about the fact that he may not be alive in six months' time (Plumb and Holland, 1974). Finally, it has been found that most adolescents, like adults, can sense that they have a terminal illness, even when they have not been told the diagnosis (Binger, p. 415). Thus, the question of whether or not to tell the patient his diagnosis is again raised.

In summary, it appears that most children over the age of four have some ability to perceive the deaths of others, but a child under the age of nine who has a terminal illness usually expresses his own "death anxiety" in terms of separation or mutilation—castration fears. It is probably not until the age of nine that the child can accurately perceive his own death and express his fears.

From this information about children's probable perceptions of death, one wonders whether any generalizations can be made about "what to tell the child." Yudkin, Kubler-Ross, Karon and Vernick, and Binger would agree that most children over the age of five should be told the truth about their terminal diagnosis, though, as Yudkin states (1967), "This aspect of the problem is the most difficult of all."

From their work with children and families, Binger et al. have written:

As parents attempted to protect their children from the concerns of the illness, children attempted similarly to protect their parents; the children who were perhaps the loneliest of all were those who were aware of their diagnosis, but at the same time recognized that their parents did not wish them to know. As a result, there was little or no meaningful communication. No one was left to whom the child could openly express his feelings of sadness, fear, or anxiety (pp. 415–416).

Although most of these authors agree that older children should be told of their diagnosis, none of them can offer a practical means of doing this. It would seem that this most difficult of problems has yet to be solved, and so most physicians wait for the child to indicate that he knows his prognosis. To quote Yudkin again (p. 40),

Can any of us, doctors, or parents, bring ourselves to do this now? Even recognizing that we are probably saving ourselves from emotional trauma by not discussing the diagnosis with the child or by lying about it, I still wonder whether it matters when we lie in this sort of circumstance.

Yudkin seems to be saying that the child will know, no matter what we say out loud.

THE PARENTS

There can be no more devastating experience in the life of a family than the fatal illness and death of a child. It tears into the family's life as a functioning unit and confronts each family member with a crisis in coping with grief and loss.

This quote from Wiener (1970) is an appropriate introduction to the subject of parents' reactions to the terminal illness of their children—reactions centering around grief over the anticipated death of the child. Bozeman et al. (1955), at the Memorial Center for Cancer and Allied Diseases in New York City, report that parents describe initial reaction to hearing the diagnosis in terms of a "physical blow to themselves." They report "it felt as if an iron safe had dropped on my head; a blow in the face," and so forth. Knudson and Natterson (1960b) report that the mothers were tense, anxious, withdrawn, and readily inclined to weep. At this point, parents want to be with their children as much as possible, and often literally cling to the child. Guilt over the child's illness is expressed aloud, as the parents search for something they might have done wrong to cause the illness (i.e., punishment). Anger and hostility are projected by parents onto the hospital or medical staff; hostility that comes from the threat of extreme loss, from the impending death of their child, and from the need to be angry at someone. Denial becomes the only feasible alternative to the parents in this early stage of grieving. The child's terminal illness poses a dramatic break in the normal parent–child relationship, and the identification of the parents with the child is so great that their pain becomes intolerable (Knudson and Natterson, 1960b).

During this first stage of what should be called "anticipatory grieving," parents are helped by associations with other parents on the wards, especially parents of terminally ill children. During this stage, parents also voice the need to learn all they can about the disease from books, doctors, and other people; to be able to ventilate their feelings to the staff without fear of judgment; and to be able themselves to provide physical care for their children. If the child should die during this first stage of the parents' adjustment, their usual reaction is hysteria, total unpreparedness for the death (Knudson and Natterson, 1960a).

When the child lives for several months after the initial diagnosis, parents begin to accept the reality of the illness and to direct their energies toward realistic measures that will help the child. They become increasingly interested in getting their children to participate in the normal activities of their environment, at home or in the hospital, and they begin to notice and to show an increasing amount of concern for sick children other than their own. Emotionally, the parents seem to be beginning to separate themselves from their dying children.

In the third and final phase of anticipatory grieving, the parents seem to show an overt calm acceptance of the fatal outcome. Knudson and Natterson (1960a) report that "there is almost no tendency to weep." In certain instances mothers express a wish that the child would die so that his suffering would be ended. Hope was expressed for children generally rather than for the mother's own child. The mother was with the child whenever possible, but with adequate consideration for the remainder of the family. There was no expression of guilt. When the children actually died, there seemed to be a mixed expression of calm sorrow and relief.

Thus, the three phases of anticipatory grieving, as seen in the parents of terminally ill children, seem to be shock and denial, depression and beginning separation from the child emotionally, and acceptance. Although this is the usual sequence of stages, many parents reach acceptance only to have their child go into a remission. When this occurs, the parent is understandably pushed back into the stage of denial, and the whole process begins again.

Parents have described several sets of conditions as helpful. The most important condition for all parents was a good relationship with their doctor. Parents need to feel that the doctor is concerned about their reactions and that he will help them with decisions. Parents express the need to talk to the doctor about when, how, and if they should tell their child of his disease, and how they should tell the child's siblings and other relatives. Friedman et al. (1963) described parents as surrounded by "concentric circles of disbelief." That is, the more distant the friend or relative, the greater that person's need to deny the illness of the child; hence, they were unable to offer real support to the parents. Because of this study, many doctors now advise parents to mention the diagnosis only to the immediate family.

In addition to needing support from their doctors, parents report receiving a great deal of support from the parents of other terminally ill children. To one author, this fact suggests that "parents' groups" might be helpful to some families; such groups are already in existence in some medical centers (Altman, 1970). Tangible help from friends with transportation, housekeeping, and baby-sitting is also reported as much needed by the parents (Bozeman et al., p. 18). It seems that such help is provided readily in the early stages of the child's illness, but as time wears on friends wear out, and the parents are left to struggle alone.

Does religion offer parents support during this time? Friedman et al. (p. 620) seem to be the only researchers who have investigated this extensively. They found that, although many parents used the church and no one left the church, few parents were able to talk in religious terms about their experiences.

Finally, after the child's death, many parents seem to appreciate the opportunity to return to the hospital or the doctor who treated the child. Binger (p. 418) has reported that, on such occasions, parents should be encouraged to discuss their reactions to the child's death and any current stresses. Such interviews or discussions seem to help the parents toward a healthy resolution of their grief.

THE NURSE

Kubler-Ross (1969) has mentioned that nurses have been the most helpful and open of the medical staff she has worked with in her interviews and seminars with dying patients. In caring for the terminally ill child, the nurse has a greater opportunity than anyone else on the medical staff to get to know the child and his family, for she is the one who is actually giving care in most situations. If nurses avoid the dying child, literally or figuratively, then that child is bound to feel very alone; but if the nurse can accept the child and his diagnosis, and work with and listen to him, she can do much to allay the child's and the family's anxieties. If she is to help the dying child and his family the nurse must be competent in the knowledge and the delivery of physical care; she must understand the factors influencing the reactions of the child and his family, and must be comfortable when working with terminally ill patients.

The importance of a nurse's being competent in the delivery of physical care cannot be overemphasized. To assign an inexperienced student or young graduate nurse to care for a dying child causes anxiety on two levels: the nurse is anxious, fearing that she will not know how to give the proper care and that the patient will know this; and she is quite liable to be anxious in the face of death. Under these circumstances, the nurse often has a totally anxiety-producing experience with the patient, and she is left feeling incompetent to deal with dying children, when she is actually unfamiliar only with the physical care involved (Quint, 1967). On the other hand, a nurse familiar with and able to provide physical care can separate her anxieties about death from the anxieties about physical care and can thus focus on learning to deal with the psychological stress death creates. Whoever assigns the neophyte nurse to care for a terminally ill child without assistance is doing both the nurse and the child a great disservice.

When the nurse is able to provide competent physical care, she must also understand the reasons for the behavior she will see in the child and his family. A nurse lacking experience with dying children is liable to assume that the quiet child is not interested in his illness, rather than that he is depressed about his condition. Or the child who is constantly calling for the nurse may be labeled as "spoiled," rather than as fearful of being alone. Parents' behavior is also easily misinterpreted by the uninformed nurse. The parent who clings to his child constantly is seen as weak and indulgent, instead of as one in the first stages of anticipatory grieving and desperately frightened of losing his child. Illustrations of behaviors that can be easily misinterpreted are endless, and the nurse who works with terminally ill children has an obligation to study the available literature on reactions to terminal illness if she is to be of any help to the child and his family.

When the nurse is a competent bedside practitioner, and when she understands the reactions of children and parents facing death, can she then work effectively and optimally with these families? The answer must be an unqualified "No." Only when she has herself learned to work comfortably with dying patients and their families—to perhaps even "enjoy" such work—is she able to function optimally with the family facing the death of a child.

How can a nurse learn to feel comfortable in the face of death? Like other medical professionals, she has probably entered the healing profession with a great deal of anxiety about death, perhaps hoping on some unconscious level to become less vulnerable to death through her work with it (Feifel, 1959; Folta, 1965). In most instances, moreover, nursing students have had little or no contact with death, so that the culture of the school they attend and its affiliated hospital have greatly influenced their attitudes (Quint, p. 6).

Quint (pp. 113–226) discusses at length how students' experiences with death can be structured and supervised to provide maximal, positive learning experiences. Two provocative suggestions are that students should have faculty role models who themselves are comfortable with dying patients and that students need a block of time, spread over their years in school, when they can come together in small seminars with qualified faculty members to discusss their changing feelings and attitudes about death.

These suggestions apply as well to the child and the family. In other words the terminally ill child and his family need a role model who is himself comfortable with death and dying, and they need time, spread over the length of the illness, to discuss their changing feelings and attitudes about the impending death. If the nurse has had an opportunity to work through her own feelings, she is the one ideal person on the medical staff who can act as such a role model. Through her efforts, time may be provided throughout the child's illness for the family to discuss their feelings with her, with the doctor, and with other parents.

SUMMARY

The nurse working with terminally ill children has perhaps the most difficult of all tasks: that of doing everything possible to allay a dying child's fears and anxieties so that he may die without feeling alone or unloved. The nurse must often step aside and let the family care for the child, focusing her support and care on them so that they can help the child through this experience. But to avoid the reality of death, with the pain and suffering it causes, is to avoid exposure to some of the most meaningful experiences human beings can have, and this is as true for nurses as it is for children, their families, and their doctors.

REFERENCES

Altman, L. 1970. "Leukemia's Impact on Family Studied." *New York Times* (March 23): p. 16.

Binger, C. M. et al. 1969. "Childhood Leukemia." *New England Journal of Medicine* 289, no. 8 (February 28):415.

Bowlby, J. 1960. "Grief and Mourning in Infancy and Early Childhood." *Psychoanalytic Study of the Child* 15:22–28.

Bozeman, M. et al. 1955. "Psychological Impact of Cancer and Its Treatment." *Cancer* 8, no. 1:18.

Feifel, H. 1959. *The Meaning of Death,* p. 122. New York: McGraw-Hill.

Fishman, K. 1968. "A Death in the Family." *New York Times Magazine* (February 11): p. 66.

Folta, J. 1965. "Perception of Death." *Nursing Research* 14 (Summer): 234.

Friedman, S. et al. 1963. "Behavioral Observations on Parents Anticipating the Death of a Child." *Pediatrics* 32 (October):618.

Furman, R. 1964. "Death and the Young Child." *Psychoanalytic Study of the Child* 19:331.

Karon, M. and J. Vernick. 1965. "Who's Afraid of Death on a Leukemia Ward?" *American Journal of Diseases of Children* 109 (May):396.

Kastenbaum, R. 1959. "Time and Death in Adolescence." In *The Meaning of Death,* ed. H. Feifel, p. 99 New York: McGraw-Hill.

———— 1969. "The Child's Understanding of Death." In *Explaining Death of Children,* ed. E. Grollman, p. 94 Boston: Beacon Press.

Knudson, A. and J. Natterson. 1960a. "Participation of Parents in the Hospital Care of Fatally Ill Children." *Pediatrics* 26 (September):484.

———— 1960b. "Observations Concerning Fear of Death in Fatally Ill Children and Their Mothers." *Psychosomatic Medicine* 22, no. 6 (June): 462.

Kubler-Ross, E. 1969. *On Death and Dying.* New York: Macmillan.

LeShan, L. 1969. "Psychotherapy and the Dying Patient." In *Death and Dying,* ed. L. Pearson, p. 46 Cleveland: Case Western Reserve University Press.

Marlow, D. 1969. *Textbook of Pediatric Nursing* (3rd ed.), p. 76 Philadelphia: W. B. Saunders Company.

Morrisey, J. R. 1965. "Death Anxiety in Children with a Fatal Illness." In *Crisis Intervention,* ed. H. Parad, pp. 324–28 New York: Family Services Association of America.

Nagy, M. 1959. "The Child's View of Death." In *The Meaning of Death,* ed. H. Feifel, pp. 88–96 New York: McGraw-Hill.

Plumb, M. and J. Holland. 1974. "Cancer in Adolescents: The Symptom Is the Thing." In *Anticipatory Grief,* ed. B. Schoenberg et al., pp. 193–209. New York: Columbia University Press.

Quint, J. 1967. *The Nurse and the Dying Patient,* pp. 19–48 New York: Macmillan.

Richmond, J. and H. Waisman. 1955. "Psychologic Aspect of Management of Children with Malignant Diseases." *American Journal of Diseases of Children* 89 (January):42–47.

Waechter, E. 1971. "Children's Awareness of Fatal Illness." *American Journal of Nursing* 71, no. 6 (June):1168–72.

Wiener, J. 1970. "Reaction of the Family to the Fatal Illness of a Child." In *Loss and Grief: Psychological Management in Medical Practice,* ed. B. Schoenberg et al., pp. 87–101. New York: Columbia University Press.

Yudkin, S. 1967. "Children and Death." *Lancet* 1 (January 7):39.

4

The Nurse's Responsibilities

A. BARBARA COYNE

It is the nurse's responsibility to help the dying person live until the moment of his death. Too often, by being labeled "terminal," the dying person is reduced to the lowest common denominator of being. Since neither the patient nor the nurse can grow in an environment of human reduction, both are diminished as individuals. Growth can occur only in an atmosphere of mutual respect for each other's humanness.

A nurse has the opportunity to know her clients well, since she spends more time with them than most other health workers do. Challenged by the reduced status of the terminal patient and its effects on all closely related family members, the nurse must assume responsibility for two interrelated areas: (1) helping the client to live until he dies and (2) helping the family to repattern its relationships and activities.

HELPING THE CLIENT LIVE UNTIL HE DIES

The nurse has many options when caring for a dying patient. In her assessment of the person who is dying, some of the nurse's responsibilities might encompass discussion of the meaning of life and death for patient and family, provision for relief of pain and for comfort, and exploration with the patient of available alternatives for treatment and care. A plan of care is included below as a demonstration.

An important aspect of the nurse's responsibility is the way in which she prepares herself to give care to the dying person. It is important not only that she investigate theories about death (including grief and bereavement), but also that she examine honestly her own feelings about life and death. Inherent in the investigation of life is investigation of the way in which the nurse views humanity. It is important to see each person as a whole individual, as a reality other than and greater than the sum of his constituent parts, in accordance with Menninger's holistic concept (1963). It is important to formulate a plan of care for each person based on individualization through the nursing process.

As humans, we derive our uniqueness from our status as rational beings: we have the ability to think, to reason, and to make judgments. We are whole, integrated beings who enjoy freedom of choice and who bear the responsibility for and the consequences of our choices. We and our environment are co-constituted, and both change and grow through this encounter. We continuously make judgments about ourselves and our environment based on the facts and information available to us as well as on our personal perception of a situation. Perceptual discriminations differ as a function of the many variables involved in living our lives. Because each of us is unique, we react wholly to a situation according to our own perceptual evaluation of it.

When a person becomes ill, it is imperative that his individuality be preserved to affirm his humanness. It is important that he continue to take part in decisions that affect his person. The nurse can provide him with some of the tools of decision making, such as relevant information about the probable consequences of alternate possible choices available to him as well as support and acceptance of the choices he makes.

It becomes clear, then, that the nurse's philosophy of life, her view of man, and her philosophy of nursing profoundly influence the way she practices nursing. Whereas the nurse must make judgments about the care of her clients, it is important for her to examine the way she arrives at these judgments. If, indeed, she believes humanity is composed of free and responsible individuals, the inferences she makes are validated by the client and, together, they identify the diagnoses. In this way he becomes an integral part of the nursing process.

Variables Affecting the Care of Dying People

We might conceive of dying people as a subcultural group, and as such, invested with the rights and responsibilities of the larger cultural group—the living. The fact of their dying should not engender attitudes of rejection or imply nonhuman status, for they are living even as they are dying: it is only that, on the spiral of life, they are predictably closer to death than some others are. Or perhaps, the distinction more accurately would be that they are cognitively closer to their death than some others.

In accepting the fact of death, nurses (and other health workers) find that they need to confront their own finiteness. Each person who dies reminds the nurse of her own fragile mortality. Until she faces the potential crisis of her own nonbeing, she has difficulty in supporting those in her care who are actually experiencing dying.

Another variable the nurse must confront is the atmosphere of the health institution that blatantly addresses itself to the prolongation of life. Although this is certainly a noble and necessary goal, it is also imperative that the health sciences raise this question: When does prolongation of life become prolongation of dying—with rejection of death? And perhaps, even more importantly, who should make the decision to prolong a life?

HELPING THE FAMILY REPATTERN RELATIONSHIPS AND ACTIVITIES

Throughout the client's illness, the nurse should remember that the family and client need each other. This is not the time to curtail visiting hours or in any other way keep them apart. The integrity of the family unit should be preserved so that the dying person does not feel alienated and, in effect, already dead. Just as the nurse and the client grow together in the process of the person's dying, so too, the family and client grow and lend support to each other in the face of their suffering. The family, together with the dying person, can begin to think of the repatterning of their lives. The nurse can help to activate this process and continue it once the client has died. Unfortunately, it is true in our society that, once the funeral is over, the family members are left to their own resources and must repattern their activities and restructure their lives in the midst of their mourning. There is a gap in services from the time of the funeral throughout the period of mourning that could be filled by the nurse as her role responsibilities continue to be reinterpreted and expanded.

Need for a Nonjudgmental Approach

It is a cultural directive of Western society to mourn and demonstrate grief in the face of death; nurses socialized in this tradition may have difficulty accepting the family that does not mourn. Usually, variables exist in individual situations to help explain nonmourning. In particular, two with which the nurse needs to be conversant are those of the family that may not feel the loss or that has already done its grief work.

In this era, when death most often occurs in an institution, family members can, in the separation imposed by a long illness, dissipate their grief by anticipating and rehearsing the death of the loved one. When death does come, family members fail to exhibit grief. They have already severed the ties, integrated the loss, and modified their life-style. The absence of grief and signs of mourning might shock and surprise family members as much as it does the nurse and could engender feelings of guilt in them. If the nurse is cognizant of these phenomena, she can resist assigning value judgments to this seemingly variant behavior and help the family to understand what has happened.

Illustrative Case Report

Betty S. was an attractive 34-year-old woman who enjoyed good books, good theatre, and the experience of being a wife and mother. She enjoyed writing short stories and poetry for her own pleasure and that of her family. She was the mother of two girls, aged 14 and 12. She described her marital relationship as mutually satisfying. Her household also included a 2-year-old beagle.

Betty was hospitalized on this admission for chemotherapy in the treatment of generalized cancer.

Past history included cancer of the breast for which a mastectomy had been done followed by removal of the ovaries. Some consideration had been given to further ablation of the endocrine activity when metastases to the brain and other areas became evident and treatment was limited to radiation therapy. She was, in fact, dying. The nurse who gave care to Betty made a number of inferences after collecting data. She validated these with Betty, and together they defined diagnoses, some of which were the following:

1. *Lack of knowledge relative to the extent of disease process.*
   Variables in the client identified by the nurse in making this inference:

   —frequent references to "going home"
   —unawareness of extent of metastases
   —questions about "other surgery" to stop disease
   —statement: "When I get home, I'm going to the library to read more about cancer."

The nurse verified her inference with Betty, who readily agreed that she did, in fact, lack knowledge of the extent of her disease. After much consultation with the physician and family, Betty was apprised of the extent of her illness and told that she was terminally ill.

2. *Feelings of loneliness, alienation, and changing self-concept.*
Variables:

—Betty cried frequently
—stated she wished her family could visit more often
—wondered if the staff thought her "ugly," since no one mentioned her rapidly balding head and her "skeleton" appearance (as she lost weight)
—stated that nurses did not look at her when they brought in her medications
—stated that she waited longer and longer periods for the nurses to answer her light.

Betty validated these inferences, and she and the nurse together put the following points into effect:

—secured permission for her daughters to visit so she could tell them herself about her terminal condition
—talked openly with staff about their feelings toward her
—talked with her husband about the possibility of buying an inexpensive wig
—wore her own night clothes.

3. *Pain and discomfort.*
Variables:

—facial grimaces and restlessness
—statements about pain in bones
—anxiety generated by confirmation of metastatic spread
—increasingly less relief from pain medication
—statements concerning fear of death.

These inferences were also validated by Betty; she and the nurse planned to:

—talk with the physician about a different drug or more frequent injections
—explore relaxation techniques

—freely discuss each others' feelings about the experience of death, pain, and suffering

—give her bath in the evening so that she could sleep in the morning

—talk openly with the family about their feelings.

Throughout this encounter with Betty, the nurse constantly assessed and evaluated her plan of care and made modifications as indicated, always including Betty and her family in the generation of the plan. During the two months of Betty's stay in the hospital, many recommendations were made; those described above were only a few used to demonstrate the nursing process for one specific client who was experiencing dying. As time passed, Betty became progressively weaker and more and more silent and lapsed at times into a deep sleep. She acknowledged her nurse and her family with a weak wave of her hand. The need for words was not so urgent as in the beginning of her hospitalization. With the nurse's help and support, she had already discussed her impending death and funeral with her family. She had even discussed with her husband the kind of woman she would like to be the mother of her two daughters once she was "gone."

Only one more request came from Betty: she missed her dog and wanted to see him once more. The nurse explored the feasibility of this; Betty was taken on a carrier to the lobby of the hospital, where Mr. S. was waiting with the dog. It was a touching reunion. Betty died two days later.

For approximately 11 months after Betty's death, the nurse continued to visit the S. family, helping them to activate the repatterning and restructuring of their lives.

SUMMARY

The nurse's responsibilities as examined in this article encompass a more expanded role than is usually envisioned. An open, honest encounter with the dying person as well as with the family after the actual death is proposed, as is involvement beyond the technical level of "doing" into the level of shared experience with the client and his family. It is painfully clear that the preparation of the nurse for this role is not now adequate. As nursing develops as a science, education for the professional's role in the human experience of dying must be explored more deeply and attention must be given to the preparation needed to help the nurse fulfill this role.

REFERENCES

Menninger, K. 1963. *The Vital Balance.* New York: Viking.

5

Case Report

YVONNE SINGLETARY

We cannot avoid death; we cannot forcibly remove it from our patients. But we can try to let it come easily so that during the terminal days the patient's pain may be alleviated with some experience of pleasure. How can we make dying easier for the patient? How can we share his fears and offer solace? This case report describes my role as a liaison nurse to the medical and surgical services of a general hospital. My work begins when a physician refers a case to me.

CASE REPORT

Until his admission, Mr. M. had worked for nearly 20 years as a "specialty cook" for a catering company. During this time he had never been absent or late for work. He maintained a single room but spent most of his free time with a female friend. Two older sisters lived near him, but his relationships with them were such that he had not notified them of his present illness.

The onset of this illness appeared to have been precipitated by an emotional situation that involved one of the sisters. Three weeks before hospitalization, Mr. M. had been invited to the home of one of his sisters, who made a demand upon him. When he refused to comply with the demand, she and her husband told him to leave. He cried after leaving her home, for he had anticipated that the invitation had meant his sister wanted to spend a pleasant evening with him. Feeling rejected, he spent the rest of that evening in a bar drinking.

Gradually, drinking became a nightly activity for him. It did not interfere with his work but did interfere with his long relationship with his female companion. He could not bring himself to tell her about the argument with his sister or explain his drinking, and so he avoided her.

Early one morning, while on his way to work, Mr. M. stopped in the emergency room of a large general hospital. Over the weekend he had coughed a lot and had had some chest pains. At times these had been severe, but he did not think that they were serious. When the doctors called him in for his examination, he appeared to be very anxious, kept looking at the large clock on the wall, and told them that he had to make bus and subway connections to arrive at his job on time. A tentative diagnosis of a lung mass was made, and immediate hospitalization for further evaluation and possible treatment was recommended.

When all the laboratory tests had been completed, a diagnosis of advanced cancer was made. Since Mr. M. constantly questioned the doctors about their findings, they decided to tell him the truth about his condition. Certain changes in his behavior became apparent when he was told. He took to pacing the corridors, did not socialize with other patients as he had done previously, and stopped smoking.

Mr. M., a 50-year-old black man, appeared to be younger than his stated age as he paced the hospital corridor. He was a striking figure, with a tall lean body, smooth brown skin, and a full head of evenly mixed white and black hair. He seemed to be in deep thought as he paced with his head bowed, oblivious to all nearby activity. After watching Mr. M. pace slowly to one end of the ward, a young intern joined me at the nurses' station and made some suggestions after filling me in on the details of his case. "Could you spend time talking with him? He has been told that he has lung cancer and that there's nothing we can do for him. I would like to send him home. He doesn't seem to be depressed, but he has been pacing more, like now, and I'm upset about the way he looks. See what you can find out from him."

I approached Mr. M. and introduced myself. I mentioned his pacing and tried to elicit some thoughts and feelings from him. He was evasive and guarded about his feelings. I asked what had brought him into the hospital. He described the signs and symptoms of his illness. Then he stated, "The doctor said I have an incurable disease." He would not say what the disease was, but talked around the issue and always referred to it as "incurable." I asked what incurable meant to him. He gave me a variety of meanings, "something you will always have," "there is no cure for the disease now," "doctors are still looking for a cure." Generalizing, he mentioned a few diseases he thought to be incurable, but he did not mention cancer nor did he say that one could die from an incurable disease.

Visiting with him on the following day, I again explained who I was and said that I hoped I could help him, adding that I would be available to talk with him about his illness or anything else that might be troubling him. As soon as I said this, he sighed deeply, settled back comfortably in his chair, and replied in a matter-of-fact manner, "You know, nurse, I didn't get upset when the doctor first told me I had cancer; it was some time later. I can't say exactly when, but I began to think about myself—my family. And there is just no time left to take care of so many things."

Now he began to talk freely about some of his feelings. No reference was made to the conversation we had had the day before about the "incurable disease." I encouraged him to continue to talk and did not challenge him about his earlier evasiveness. He was able to express some of his feelings, and a kind of catharsis started to take place. His depression became more apparent as he talked, but it frequently gave way to anger and pain. Finally, I announced that I would have to

leave but that I would return when he wanted me. He said he
would like me to visit with him on the next day.

Mr. M. did not pace in the corridor the next day. He
stayed in his room talking with other patients. During visiting hours he left the room to sit in an isolated end of the
ward and watch the elevator. When we met, he began the
conversation by saying he knew I was very busy and he would
understand if I could not talk with him. I assured him that I
had time to spend with him. He talked about how much better he felt since our first talk. Now we talked about cancer,
his understanding of it, and his personal thoughts and feelings about having it. "This is another injustice to me. Why
am I still being punished? No one knows what I have gone
through." He expressed the thought that the doctors were
mistaken, because his symptoms had developed so suddenly.
His smoking had been moderate, but he had been drinking
more recently to "forget." Each statement or question was
laden with emotion. He spoke freely again about cancer but
did not pursue the new issues he had raised. When he finished exploring his feelings about cancer, he was quiet for a
long period. Finally, he spoke, "Nurse, I know the doctor
still wants to discharge me, but I have no place to go, just to
my room. I'll be alone there . . . no one to talk to . . . I've
done such a lot of terrible things in my life. I don't have a
family, haven't had one for years. Those who are still living
don't want me." After another long pause, he continued, "If
the doctor could only tell me how long I have, a week or two
. . . maybe five . . . if he could just tell me!" He leaned
forward, rested his head between his hands, and said almost
in a whisper, "I don't see why I have to die alone."

Mr. M. became depressed. He still hoped the doctors were
wrong. Being in the hospital provided him with some hope
that the mistake would be corrected. Hospitalization also
provided contact with other people, something he claimed he
did not have in the outside world. There were also many
unresolved conflicts he wanted to work through or, at least,

bring into the open before he died. He was asking me for help.

After this meeting I discussed the possibility of extending Mr. M.'s hospitalization with the medical resident and the intern. I presented his current emotional status and the need to determine the nature of his depression as reasons for my request. They agreed to hold discharge plans in abeyance until further notice from me.

Mr. M. began to test my commitment to him. His adult life had been a series of one rejection after another from people who he thought cared about him. He had no reason to trust me or believe that I accepted him as a human being. I could only demonstrate my commitment and establish trust by keeping appointments and allowing him to talk freely. He began to tell me about his family, what it was like growing up in a small suburban area in a Northern state, the only son in a family of six girls, one of the few black families in the area. His family was closely knit, financially secure, and well respected by everyone. Both parents worked and insisted upon sending each child for special training after high school at a time when most black children of school age had to leave school to help support the family.

After completing trade school, he had married a woman from a family similar to his own. They were called an ideal couple. He claimed that they were very much in love, but he felt inadequate as a husband at times. Friends and neighbors were constantly telling him how lucky he was to have such a wife. His father often said he did not deserve her. These comments made him want to demonstrate to everyone his love for his wife by providing her with many material comforts. His job paid well, but he needed more money when the children began to come, and he continued to indulge his wife. Before concluding this session, he repeated several times, "If only I had a chance to do it again, it would be different." He did not go any further or say what would be different as he drifted off into deep thought.

At our fifth meeting Mr. M. began by saying, "Nurse, I'm

going to tell you something I've never told anyone. I'm not afraid of dying, we all have to die sometime . . . no, death doesn't bother me. One thing has bothered me for nearly 30 years . . . it seems to bother me more now." He said it was related to his family and began to tell some of the history. In his desire to provide the best for his wife and children, he became involved in an illegal money-making scheme. When he was caught, he found he had also violated the mores of his family and his community. He was incarcerated for a period of time as punishment and then was banished from the family for having disgraced them in his community. Even though he was an adult with a family, living away from home, his father made the decision to deprive him of his community and his family. According to his father, he had given up his rights as a son, husband, and father when he broke the law. The father's word was final. Mr. M. considered this severe punishment but accepted it and was never treated as a member of his family again, giving up his parents, his wife, his children, and his siblings. Although nearly 30 years had passed, he was still treated as if the incident were still fresh. In the beginning he was able to maintain contact with his wife and children by writing and sending money to support them. Then their letters to him stopped, and he learned that his father had assumed responsibility for his family.

He began to save his money. His siblings continued to regard him as an outcast but often asked him for financial assistance. Large sums of money borrowed from him were never repaid. He made infrequent visits to their homes, usually only when he was invited. At his father's death, he was not asked to attend the funeral, but the death did provide him with an opportunity to establish some contact with his mother. He was reduced to tears as he recalled the hell he had been going through. He spoke of loneliness and the use of alcohol to deal with depression. He talked of how his life might have been different if he had only been wise enough to make the right choice. He longed to know his children and find out what they thought of him. He did not mind dying but felt his life had been for nothing. He continued to reveal details of his life and the coping methods he had used to sustain himself. This information was given in segments during our regular daily meetings. When other patients received visitors, I visited with Mr. M., who had none. Most of the time I listened to him. These visits took place during the week but never on weekends, and he would tell me how, on weekends, he looked forward to Mondays. Each Friday he walked me to the elevator saying he would see me on Monday.

Mr. M.'s physical condition began to deteriorate. He was increasingly short of breath and required oxygen; yet, he waited anxiously for my visit and talked without using the oxygen until our hour together was over.

When we first began our visits, insomnia had been noted. He spoke of being afraid of sleep. His nights were spent sitting in a chair at a distance from his bed. Gradually, he moved his chair closer to the bed. At first he would say, "I'm just not sleepy. . . . I haven't been sleepy since the doctor said I have cancer." "Are you afraid to sleep?" I asked. After a long pause, he answered, "Yes. It's the feeling in my chest. When it gets that way, I can cough and it gets better. I can't cough if I'm sleeping, I won't be able to catch my breath. My chest gets tight at night, so I don't go near the bed."

We began to have discussions about guilt. Although he had been guilty of violating family mores, the family was also guilty of making unreasonable demands on him. We examined each situation and saw evidence of several attempts he had made to undo the wrong he had done earlier. He had established himself in a good job, saved a considerable amount of money, and was respected by his friends. As he compared the original violation to the punishment he continued to suffer, he was able to verbalize how out of proportion the latter had been to the former. He was now able to see his family in a different light and realized that they were not perfect. He also realized that they were still punishing him because he permitted it. He decided he had paid his debt off a long time ago. Then, for the first time since he had been hospitalized, he called his sisters and told them of his condition.

They advised him not to call other relatives, particularly his mother, who lived in another state, because she would only worry about him. But he did call his mother, and he also called his former wife and children. His children had married, and he learned that he was a grandfather. The children were overjoyed at hearing from him and later sent him a telegram wishing him well. At last, too, his local family came to visit with him in the hospital.

Two days later, Mr. M. greeted me with, "I'm beginning to feel sleepy. I know I will sleep tonight." I suggested that he take a nap, but he was anxious to talk to me about the first conversation he had had with his daughter in 24 years. Over the weekend relatives from out of state had made a special trip to see him and had told him that he could return home to live with his mother when he was discharged from the hospital. His female friend, informed of his illness by one of his sisters, came to visit him before our visit ended.

The next day Mr. M. seemed to be very fatigued. His chair was next to the bed. Although he had been exhausted the day before, he had not been able to sleep. Anti-anxiety medication was given as ordered by the doctor. He told me, "I have so much sleep to catch up on, I was afraid I'd miss you today if my eyes were closed." But he could hardly keep his eyes open and said, "I guess I'm not very much company for you today." I assured him that I would sit with him for one hour even if he had nothing to say. He used the oxygen a few times but did not sleep. As I prepared to leave, he asked, "Will you be back tomorrow?"

When I returned the following afternoon, he was sitting in the same position. He greeted me with a big smile. "I didn't think I could wait for you. I'm so tired, but I made it." I replied, "You do look tired today and I know you are afraid to go to sleep. I'll be with you, so why don't you relax with your head on the bed for a little while? Come on, put your head down and just relax." He placed his head on the side of his bed. Holding his oxygen mask near his face, he began to relax and breathed easily into sleep. I remained at his bedside writing a report as he slept. After about 45 minutes, I turned my attention back to him. He seemed to be sleeping, but I soon realized how still he was—that he was dead.

I studied his face for a few minutes. He looked almost happy. Death had not come as a fearful and painful thing. I pulled the curtains around his bed, walked out into the corridor, and asked the intern to go to Mr. M.

6

Continuing and Discontinuing Care

KENNETH A. CHANDLER

When asked what it was that he looked for most in those who cared for him, a dying patient replied, "Well, for someone to look as if they are trying to understand me. I'm hard to understand" (Saunders, 1969, p. 63). This *is* care that continues and is indeed the underpinning of continuing care. Unfortunately, as Strauss (1969) points out, although physicians and nursing staff * may be exceptionally capable in their technical skills, their behavior toward the patient may reflect less upon their professional training and more upon their anxieties. The resulting mode of "caring" may often be one in which the physical demands of the patient are met with as much dispatch as possible and with an increasing tendency on the part of nursing staff to lessen patient contact. This *is* discontinuing care—care that is mobilized for the momentary demand and ceases when the patient is made comfortable. Unfortunately, "making comfortable" may well refer more to the feelings of the nursing staff and less to the patient. Witness a terse chart note, "Patient given sedative and resting quietly"! The impersonal quality of staff–patient interaction, often dictated by techniques and procedures,

---

* The term *nursing staff* refers to all members of the hospital staff having contact with the patient.

contributes little, in and of itself, to the enhancement of the patients' experiencing care that continues.

It would appear that discontinuing care occurs more frequently in situations where patients are described as "chronically ill," and particularly where their illness is terminal. I have described this patient–staff interaction in an earlier paper (Chandler, 1965), where the differing behaviors of dying patients reflected coping mechanisms of the patient as well as the staff. My intent here is to extend the application of those findings to establish more meaningful relationships with those for whom sustained emotional ties have been disrupted, that is, those dying and those in the process of dissolution through chronic illnesses. Apparently, in extended contact between patient and staff, an interaction develops that is erosive to the patient's desire to continue and to the nursing staff's ability to continue to care.

With an increased life span, increased family mobility, and the greater availability and use of hospitalization, it is not surprising that an increasing number of patients come to hospitalization earlier in their chronic illnesses. For some it is clear that the medical care needed dictates their continued hospitalization, but for others their hospitalization reflects more a lack of capability to provide such care arising from emotional and physical (space) limitations. In either case, previously sustaining relationships are often disrupted, and in their place the nursing staff becomes the focus of increased dependency needs. As Verwoerdt (1964) points out, hospitalization promotes regression, and "regressed patients become egocentric, sensitive and emotionally labile"; their demands, despairs, and depressions reflect their inordinate felt *loss of someone who cares.* Physician and nurse alike become loved and feared, praised and damned, friend and foe as the patient attempts to work through his feelings of loss and loneliness. Few have been prepared to endure such a continuing emotional fusillade, and most nursing staff are vulnerable to their own reactions against such loss. Professional competency and positive self-regard slowly become eroded until the nursing staff vacillates in the tortuous relationship like a chip of wood on an angry sea. It is not surprising to find bewilderment and puzzlement on the part of the staff who are attempting to cope with the varying emotional outbursts. In the absence of assistance to the staff, one observes that their frustration and resentment emerge as an increase in authoritarianism, displacement, and rejection. On the other hand, patients become more and more disruptive or flee to withdrawal in the presence of their increased feelings of helplessness. Such then is the situation when care is discontinued and in its place both patient and staff come to care less.

It has been my privilege over the past several years to spend a good deal of time with dying patients, groups of those chronically ill, and nursing staff who care for them in both private and public hospitals. The dedication of many to providing such care is indeed impressive; the expressions of helplessness on the part of both patient and staff are similarly notable. It becomes clear to me that, in the care of those chronically ill or dying, few get better, and the care of the nursing staff appears to diminish in its significance in the presence of the fact of death. The traditional goals of therapeutic care no longer hold, and often patients who have, indeed, been cared for are seen to become debilitated. If, as Norton (1963) states, "the crucial gift of the therapist is that of himself . . . to enable the patient to defend against loss," what resource is available to the nursing staff to enable them to withstand the repetitive loss that is so much a part of *their* day-to-day experience? What sustains the therapist who treats the dying? Perhaps the answer may be more poignantly seen in the words of a patient who handed me the following poem she had written:

> To be
> Is to be with;
> To be with
> Is to be

In a sense it would seem that this means to be able to experience with the patient his experiences of himself, or as Rogers wrote, "to perceive the world as the client sees it, to communicate empathic understanding" (1951, p. 29). It is my impression that this aspect of patient care is most neglected in the training of nursing staff. Those who are to engage in continuing care, both physician and nurse, need to be assisted in coming to grips with their own vulnerabilities. As Coleman (1962, p. 3) has said, "It is important . . . to learn how to deal usefully with [one's] own disturbed reactions to . . . evocative behavior of the patient" and to realize that the patient needs "to play out his ambivalent conflicts in such a way as to involve the other person as deeply as possible" (p. 2).

In my early contacts with continuing-care hospitals, it became apparent that the many referrals for me to see patients reflected more a request for help from the staff rather than psychopathology on the part of the patient. Often the need for tranquilizers or sedatives arose from a particular patient–staff interaction rather than from some deep-seated intrapsychic disturbance. Similarly conspicuous was the desire of both patient and staff for a situation in which they could talk about each other or with each other and reflect their disquietudes or often just ask that something be done about this or that. With this in mind, regular group meetings were established, sometimes separately, sometimes jointly, with staff and patients. Described below are some of the major issues with which the members of these groups have been concerned rather consistently over the past several years; to the extent that these issues became less emotionally charged for members of both groups, they became less the focal point for manipulation and disruption of a more positive nursing-staff–patient interaction.

1. Feelings of Helplessness

Patients often saw themselves as helpless and in turn demanded more help from the nursing staff. The nursing staff similarly felt helpless to deal with their patients' helplessness. Both felt insecure in their expectations of each other. Nursing staff were often ill at ease in the presence of emotional outbursts, for example, crying, anger, or protracted silence; patients were irritated at even reasonable delays to their requests. As Verwoerdt pointed out, for both, helplessness reflected their loss of self-confidence. As they were able to examine their feelings in this respect, viewing them in terms of a reality anchor, they became more at ease in making reasonable demands and having realistic expectations.

This is a continuing process, sensitive to changes in the patient's disease and to the varying vulnerabilities of both. To this date such issues continue to recur and reflect continued caring.

2. Feelings Concerning Privacy

Patients do indeed realize that hospitalization implies they will be examined, studied, observed, and asked innumerable questions. Many feel that everyone knows everything and that there is little opportunity for privacy. Nursing staff are said to enter rooms whose doors are closed without knocking, and often some physicians walk behind a curtained patient without notice. More serious perhaps is the feeling that there is no opportunity for a shared confidence to remain confidential! Ambivalence on the part of both patient and nursing staff leads them to errors of judgment about what is private and what is a proper concern. Sexual matters often pose difficulties for both.

As both were able to discuss aspects of privacy, become reacquainted with rights and responsibilities of each, changes were effected in this area of felt neglect. However, it is clear that in a long-term continuing relationship, much becomes taken for granted and is reflected by the frequency with which this topic emerges in both groups.

3. Feelings of Neglect

This is an area of particular concern to many patients, and their concern is reflected in the attitudes of nursing staff. Physicians, family, and nurses often feel insecure in the presence of the dying, the paralyzed, and the middle-aged stroke patient and tend to avoid them. Some patients rarely have visitors; some are seen very infrequently by their physicians and then often very briefly; some, because they demand less care, have little contact with the nursing staff. Patients who expressed feelings of being neglected the most were not in fact so neglected. Such feelings were often found to reflect feelings of resentment and anger over their situations or to mirror depressive features coming to the fore. Nursing staff often expressed negative attitudes toward families of such patients and frequently "felt sorry" for them; in some instances nursing staff made special efforts on these patients' behalf. In some instances it was clear that the anger of the nursing staff toward families was a displacement of anger toward the patient for making such demands.

The role of adequate social service and volunteer groups becomes clearly important as a buffer for this inadvertent neglect. However, it was noted that, as patients in the group slowly began to form ties within the group or with a particular individual, *felt neglect* was lessened, even though some aspects of real neglect were not changed.

4. Unrealistic Expectations

Frequently the expectations of patients about their own illnesses reflected more their hopes than the reality. For some, miracles "could still happen," and for others there was little realization that their illness set the stage for the relative permanency of hospitalization. This area posed the greatest challenge for the patient group; occasionally a patient left the group as realistic appraisal by group members became intolerable, but he often returned with less bitterness and more strength to cope with the fact of his illness. Much time was spent in discussing the limitations existing and expected from various diseases. Patients often knew more about their condition than they revealed in usual conversation. Continuing pressure from the patient group for increased information on the many illnesses represented was observed. This was seen to shift from a simple curiosity to serious attempts to understand what the course of a particular disease might be; in many instances patients became less emotionally distraught about their condition as they understood it more fully.

The nursing staff, similarly, were not altogether certain about what they might expect from particular patients. Often their value judgments of a patient's behavior overlooked specific clinical knowledge that was undoubtedly available in their training, certainly available in the medical library, but for complex reasons was not accessible in their day-to-day decision making. This was particularly the case for patients who seemed to be physically capable (not paralyzed) but were stabilized from traumatic brain damage or for those who were slowly deteriorating from a degenerative disease. The nursing staff were often not cognizant of the implications of cerebral damage for impulsive behavior, memory deficits, and the more subtle disruptions in logical thinking.

Continuing discussions are indeed important to enable the nursing staff to realize that disagreeable behavior may be as much a symptom of the illness as the disease itself (Verwoerdt, 1964). In this respect, continuing assessment of patients' status and of changes is essential so that the nursing staff can shift both their attitudes and demands toward their patients. Special consideration needs to be given to the behavior of mentally retarded patients.

5. Crying, Silence, and Depression

Perhaps there are few behavioral manifestations that create a greater feeling of helplessness among the nursing staff than those of crying, silence, and depression. It is as if in their presence one indeed becomes impotent. In discussions of these aspects of behavioral change, feelings of anger, sympathy, resentment, intolerance, and disgust were revealed. Both the nursing staff and patients alike felt compelled to "do something"—though they were never quite certain about what to do. Frequently, psychological/psychiatric consultation was sought; the interpretations of such behavior by both groups reflected their many differing value systems. To do nothing in the presence of crying or silence seemed to them intolerable; it became clear that the disquietudes of the staff demanded and led to inappropriate actions. This area was one that was most fruitful for attitude change, evoking much feeling and providing many opportunities for self-examination.

As the staff became more at ease with their feelings of being unable to cope with crying or silence, they found that light teasing and banter enabled them to communicate their acceptance to the patient. It seemed that, as they became able to be with a patient in silence, the nursing staff became more confident of being able to communicate more meaningfully.

While other issues and other concerns became important from time to time for both patients and the nursing staff, those presented here seem to exemplify the needs of both to share their anxieties, perceive more clearly the feelings of others, and by so doing, develop a greater sense of adequacy. The day-to-day interaction of patient and nursing staff in a continuing-care relationship is such as to mobilize defenses continually against feelings of inadequacy on the part of both. As withdrawal occurs and patient contact decreases, *continuing care is discontinued,* and in its place there emerges *care that is chronic,* and with it a less-than-caring attitude on the part of both patient and staff. In the continuing-care relationship a greater demand is placed on the self-identity of the nurse than on her technical competence. On a day-to-day basis she must sustain a relationship that contributes to the therapeutic milieu of the patient. The vicissitudes of such a demand for continuing care have been presented here. To avoid the emergence of care that is chronic and the discontinuance of caring, it was found that increased opportunities for viewing oneself and others in the caring relationship effected more nearly adequate coping for both nurse and patient and significantly buffered the erosion of caring.

REFERENCES

Chandler, K. A. 1965. "Three Processes of Dying and Their Behavioral Effects." *Journal of Consulting Psychology* 29:296–301.

Coleman, J. 1962. "Banter as Psychotherapeutic Intervention." *American Journal of Psychoanalysis* 22:1–6.

Norton, J. 1963. "Treatment of a Dying Patient." In *The Psychoanalytic Study of the Child*, ed. R. S. Eissler. New York: International Universities Press 28:541–60.

Rogers, C. 1951. *Client-Centered Therapy.* New York: Houghton Mifflin.

Saunders, C. 1969. "The Moment of Truth: Care of the Dying Patient." In *Death and Dying*, ed. L. Pearson. Cleveland: Case Western Reserve University Press.

Strauss, A. L. 1969. "Family and Staff During Last Weeks and Days of a Terminal Illness." *Annals of the New York Academy of Sciences* 164 (December): 687–95.

Verwoerdt, A. 1964. "Communication with the Fatally Ill." *Journal of the Southern Medical Association* 57:787–95.

ADDITIONAL BIBLIOGRAPHY

Weisman, A. D. 1970. "Misgivings and Misconceptions in the Psychiatric Care of Terminal Patients." *Psychiatry* 33(1):67–81.

Weisman, A. D. and T. P. Hackett. 1961. "Predilection to Death." *Psychosomatic Medicine* 23:232–55.

7

A Case Review on Death, from Two Perspectives

JOAN M. LIASCHENKO
and
RICHARD J. TORPIE

Both of us entered into a unique relationship during the past year—that of a physician—radiation oncologist (RT) with a self-perpetuated long-term interest in thanatology and no other particular qualifications to act as a preceptor for a registered nurse (JL), turned mental health technologist, who would spend an internship year working with dying patients. Many of these patients were on other services, and we could act only as participant–observers, only slightly bending personal and institutional attitudes that existed firmly and sometimes brutally with regard to the care of patients with malignant terminal illness. As health professionals we had learned the talent of empathy, the moderately deep identification with the patient and his needs, that can usually be turned off at five o'clock and that protects the care given from emotional devastation. Yet more and more with regard to terminal illness, we found the qualities of empathy and appropriate responses strained by lack of support of the emotional needs of the care given, by the depersonalization of the patient by barriers in communications, and by the absence of emotional support for the patient as he faced the onslaught of repeated therapeutic failures.

This report then is in the form of a diary describing the last few days in the life of a young man. One of us describes comments from a deep supporting role to the patient, the other, somewhat from the periphery, where surrounding events could be observed.

RT: I first saw his X-ray, a barium swallow of the esophagus, that showed erosion and stiffening of that entire structure from what could be leukemic or infectious infiltrate. A resident passing by commented expressively with an ominous whistle and a very negative shaking of the head. Of course, the thin and huddled figure in the sheets on the litter behind us could then see the professional confirmation of how wretched he felt.

I examined Jay, who was in his early twenties. He was in a leukemic relapse, despite aggressive and skilled drug therapy. His reason for a radiation therapy referral was the agonizing mediastinal pain he experienced whenever he swallowed, even his saliva. I did my best to reassure him that radiation should bring relief within two or three days. This was all I could offer as a physician, and I felt relieved that he was not my primary patient. This clue within myself and the desolateness of the person in front of me made me feel that he could benefit from a thanatology consultation.

JL: Jay was a young college student dying of leukemia. His diagnosis had been established nine months previously on a visit to the student-health center at an upstate university, after a week of vague symptoms. A blood test was done immediately, and he was promptly and bluntly told that he had leukemia. After establishment of the diagnosis, he experienced a somewhat poor clinical course for three months, at which time a remission occurred, lasting for six months until this relapse for acute lymphocytic leukemia. His primary management was by the medical oncologists, but now his bone marrow had failed because of his disease, and this limited appropriate chemotherapy. The reason he offered for this admission was "that his blood count was low."

I met with him four days after admission, on the advice of Dr. Torpie. He was 24 years old, pale, frail, and thin. He was bald as a result of chemotherapy. His private room was strewn with soda cans, unfinished plastic model kits, and reading material. He was restless and exhibited much overt anxiety; he occasionally paced the room and fidgeted. He was quite rational, but his speech was pressured by the exertion of his condition. He was eager to talk and explained how he would organize his day in the hospital. He expressed some self-recrimination. "My family would do anything for me and look what they got, a bum!" His mood was depressed with anxious but appropriate affect. He jumped from subject to subject, rushing his thoughts, and it was difficult for me to keep up with this diffuse conversation. Aware of this, he stated that he needed to talk badly and that perhaps then he would be calmer. He was receiving Valium (10 mg. t.i.d.) and on admission had been given a stat dose of Thorazine.

This overt, anxious behavior continued for the first two interviews, which usually lasted an hour and a half. During this time, I just listened. By the third session he was remarkably less anxious, probably because of two factors. First, his more frightening symptoms of hematemesis and hemorrhaging into the cornea had subsided. For the first three days after admission Jay experienced these symptoms and was terrified, for he was in a private room far removed from the nurse's station. The nurses, he felt, were not answering his calls quickly enough. To help alleviate Jay's terror, his older brother had come from home, two hours away, and stayed with him, sleeping at night in a chair. When Jay's symptoms had subsided and he felt able to cope with the hospitalization, his brother returned home. By now, a relationship between us had been established that enabled him to ventilate his anxiety. Jay was from a city in northern Pennsylvania and did not receive visitors regularly.

RT: After three treatments with radiation therapy much of his pain was relieved, but I noted new bleeding points under the skin and several nodules that represented leukemic infiltration. He began expressing hope for a remission and ascribed more potential to the radiation therapy regarding control of his disease than was possible. I tried to modulate his expectations without showing agreement but also without poking a hole in his balloon. The likelihood of any remission was quite remote.

JL: After the overt anxiety diminished, Jay and I discussed ways hospitalization could be made better for persons with leukemia and cancer. I frequently ask this question because it is helpful to me as a student thanatologist and it also provides a gentle and effective tool. Many sessions with Jay were tape recorded, and he enjoyed doing this. As a fellow classmate commented, perhaps this provided him with a sense of immortality. She was probably correct, for Jay was informed that the tapes would be kept intact. Within this frame of reference Jay was able to talk about dying and death. Two things were most important to him: first, that there be someone such as myself to talk with these patients and, second, that leukemia and cancer patients be placed on the same floor with a regular patient's group for support.

At this point, Jay was able to talk about his feelings when his disease was first diagnosed. He related that after he was informed he felt as if he would die shortly, since all leukemia is fatal. He described these first few hours as utter confusion; his thoughts were racing, but he couldn't organize them. The student-health physician suggested that Jay contact his family physician, and Jay did so immediately. After informing the doctor of his diagnosis, Jay said, "Doc, how are we going to tell mom?" Much support was given by the family physician, who then relayed the information to Jay's mother. That night Jay returned to his apartment, where friends had gathered. The concern of his friends impressed Jay. "Funny," he said, "how my friends took the news according to how they lived from day to day." One stated in a blasé fashion "that we all have to go sometime." Another passed out quarts of beer, used a cigarette to burn a hole in a piece of plastic, and then smoked a "joint." He was unable to say anything. But another friend said very optimistically that you're going to be fine because they cure all leukemia. For Jay this was most helpful, for he described it as a transition from resignation to fight. By the following morning Jay felt confident that he would "beat this thing."

One day while discussing patient groups, I mentioned that some people, although not all, died from leukemia. Jay turned rather abruptly and calmly stated that he didn't know that. Somewhat nonchalantly he added that it was "kind of scary." Here I pointed out that at this time last year he had thought that all leukemia is fatal. People died of leukemia, he said, only because of complications, which he defined as infections. When I questioned him on his difficulty with swallowing, he responded that it was a result of overeating.

We spent many hours talking religion and Jay's philosophy of life in general. Jay was a vibrant, alive person whose worldly desires consisted of becoming a history professor at a small college, getting married, and raising a family. But his ever-increasing doubts were present as he asked, "Is that asking too much?" Although not practicing Roman Catholicism, into which he had been born and raised, Jay had deep religious convictions. He believed in a spirit, though perhaps not a God, as Catholics are taught. Eternity or the concept of an afterlife was more doubtful to him. "If there is one, however," he said, "I will ask God or this Spirit to judge me on the fact that I searched for the truth."

RT: After the fifth day of treatment his pain was relieved, and I had to make a decision on continuation of therapy. His laboratory reports worsened, and he required fresh blood and platelets. He decided for me, stating he "wanted to go on with this thing."

JL: Hope is a most abstract term that occurs constantly in the literature on dying persons. In a conversation one day, the topic arose. After a few minutes of thought, Jay said, "Hope is the ability to fulfill oneself as one is." The beauty and humanness of his definition greatly impressed me. Avery

Weisman (1972), a Harvard psychiatrist with much experience with dying persons, has defined hope as "having confidence in the desirability of survival." The similarity between the two statements intrigued me. In an attempt to be more specific about his definition, he admitted that hope was another six-month remission, after which he would, of course, return for another course of chemotherapy.

"Hope," Weisman says, "arises from a desirable self-image, healthy self-esteem, and a belief in our ability to exert a degree of influence on the world surrounding us." These would be exactly the qualities that eventually enabled Jay to overcome his fears of death and die in peace with dignity. In discussing the formulation, I address myself to his guilt, his use of denial, and object loss through death.

Guilt reactions are common in patients with cancer and other malignant diseases. Jay's guilt, I think, originated from his fantasies of his mother's reaction to his death. He was the youngest of four children, and his father had died when Jay was 12. When his mother and brother returned from the hospital bearing his father's clothes, he remembered feeling terribly sad and being unable to understand why. Jay described his mother's reactions to her husband's death as "hysterical." She cried for months, and it was painful to watch her. An uncle, to whom Jay had grown particularly close after his father's death, died in March 1971. On the night of the viewing, Jay's mother suffered an angina attack for which she was hospitalized. Jay attributed this to his uncle's death, and his memory of his mother's experience frightens him. If he should die, what would happen to her? Perhaps my own anxiety interfered with Jay's expressing this more overtly. He never spoke of this in a direct way.

Kubler-Ross (1969) has defined stages of dying that have served as helpful guidelines, although she implies that they are static entities that follow a logical sequence, and this implication has limited our total view of the patient. Weisman states, "Denial is present throughout terminal illness in various degrees depending upon the patient's deployment of defenses, his physical condition, and changes in his psychosocial field," which are phases of personal responses to the course of fatal illness. Much of Jay's anxiety was handled by vacillating between denial and acceptance, a common, if not essential, response in fatal illness. The French writer de la Rochefoucauld (in Wahl, 1959), said, "just as one cannot always look at the sun, so also one cannot always look at death." The complete reversal from knowing he would die to saying that only those with complications die served as a much-needed defensive measure that enabled him to fight his disease and not submit to despair.

By denying that his dysphagia was a complication, Jay demonstrated second-order denial. Weisman lists three levels of denial: first order—denial of the disease itself; second order—denial of the implications of the disease; and third order—denial of death itself.

During the three weeks that I saw Jay, he was experiencing middle knowledge, which Weisman defines as an area of uncertain certainty. It lies somewhere between open acceptance of one's death and its utter repudiation. Thus Jay was able to talk about death, albeit in a philosophical way. Both of us talked of Jay's going home again. Perhaps I believed it much more than he did. Although I had been reading the chart, the serious implications of the medical language were simply not registering.*

Jay was going to die and thereby lose all "object relations," a thought that was the primary source of his anxiety. Not until my experience with dying people had that term held any real meaning for me. Now it is the very essence of dying and my work. It is difficult for most people to imagine the feeling of having one's contact with others, especially loved ones, slip away. Soon there will be no one, and the person will be completely and forever isolated. It is a terrifying thought, and for the dying patient it is a reality. Janice Nor-

* It may be that we were participating in a conspiracy that would save us both from the sorrow we would feel. To participate in the dying of one your own age transforms the idea of death into a frightening reality.

ton (1963), a psychoanalyst, defines the major problem of the dying person as object loss. A therapist helps the dying patient by defending against this loss. In technical analytic terms I could not describe how I accomplished this, or even, in fact, be sure that I did. I know, however, that I was helpful, although I did nothing profound. I was simply there.

RT: The last of Jay's reserve was vanishing. I had stopped therapy to the esophagus; his discomfort in swallowing was returning. He pointed to some slightly painful swelling in the scrotum, which I realized would become a major problem with leukemia infiltration, but I elected to hold off therapy unless absolutely needed. He indicated that he had lost interest in his models, as if sensing they would never be completed, and also in his books, which would never be read. He talked of the possibility of returning to school if he had a remission, and he told me how he had considered law or history, but he let the matter drift when I could not reply to his concept of future life. My thoughts began to wander. I could think about my weekend off and pleasures of late summer. I thought of my two-year-old child and wished she would never experience what Jay was now living through. I thought of flowerbeds that must be turned for the winter. I thought of Jay's love of life.

JL: Starting with the following quote by Weisman, I would like to share with the reader my experience of participation in Jay's dying and death: "We grow up with the assistance of the monuments, tools, writing, mementoes of those who lived before us. We can also enhance the meaning of being alive by touching the edge of life that is slipping away."

On Friday, September 15, Jay was again suffering from dysphagia, which had increased over the past few days. Because of my expectations I was totally unprepared for what I faced on Monday. It was 2:00 P.M., much later than our usual appointment, when I read the progress notes, as was my customary procedure. Under the date were listed numerous, ominous physical signs and symptoms. Among them were a temperature of 103.6, perirectal absess, and gangrenous buttocks. As I scanned the note, I became totally oblivious to these data and recognized only the words "poor prognosis" that screamed out from this page. The reality of the words was, however, incongruent with my thoughts. With the idea that he must be sicker than I was aware, I started toward the room as if my usual cheerful self. Jay was usually vibrant and alive to himself and the world around him. He possessed the gift of inspiring people to feel, act, and be in love with life. As I entered his room, a pale, sickly face enveloped in stark white sheets turned toward me. Quickly my eyes darted around the room, only to locate a "crash box," intravenous fluids, and a hypothermia machine. After a few minutes of adjusting to this "technological darkness," I moved to the side of the bed, where I acknowledged the reality by saying that things didn't look very well. With an expression full of fright, he responded that they weren't but added that I had kept our appointment.

Subsequently, Jay began talking incoherently, although I recognized his need for a nurse. In the hall I spoke with a nurse who volunteered that Jay was doing very poorly and would probably die before the day had ended. With this information I became very frightened and, at the same time, sorrowful. I had an intense need to talk with someone, and so I called Dr. Torpie, who was at another hospital. By the time he reached the phone I was crying very hard and blurted out that Jay was going to die—today. The humanness and concern of Dr. Torpie's immediate response—"Is he alone?"—was probably a major factor in my subsequent ability to handle my feelings and be of help to Jay. But because I was still obviously too distraught to be of any help, Dr. Torpie suggested I return to the office and wait for him so that we could see Jay together. I agreed, but as I returned the receiver to the phone, I was bombarded by feelings. A nurse handed me a box of tissues, and I became acutely aware of my guilt and embarrassment for crying, especially at a busy nursing station. As I moved to a less conspicuous place, "Is he alone?" became paramount in my feelings. Suddenly I realized that it wasn't bad or silly to cry, but if I was unable to gain control over myself, then I must definitely think about selecting another area in which to work.

RT: I realized this was a crisis for her of the greatest dimensions. She had gone beyond the limits of empathy and was now caught up in the whirlwind of compassion, in its oldest meaning and identification—a fellowship in suffering between equals. In a sense she was dying. After three months of experience and observations with dying patients she was not totally caught up with reality. I was afraid she needed support, but I also knew two hours separated Jay from his nearest relatives, and now, at least, he could have someone who was close. The experience of this involvement must be suffered. It would be her "baptism under fire" and strengthen her in all other future experience with dying patients, or it could "turn her off," depending on her supervisor's handling of identification or countertransference.

JL: Within five minutes, I was composed and I returned to Jay. During the next hour, I sat by the bedside attempting to comfort him. Jay was in agonizing pain, but no further narcotics were given. Although delirious, he communicated his desire to have the pain removed. It is difficult to watch someone suffer and be impotent to alleviate their sufferings. I could not relieve his pain, but I assured him that I would remain with him. At the end of the hour Jay lifted himself to the side of the bed. This action gave me the intense feeling that he wanted me to take him in my arms. I psychologically pulled away and was unable to hold him. How I resent my behavior. I probably denied him his last earthly wish—to be held as a person, not a patient, by another person, not a staff member.

As Jay dropped to the pillow, respiratory distress began. I rang for the nurses. Within seconds, three nurses had answered the call and became very busy. Moving to the side of the bed, I took his hand. Nestled among busy people and things, I talked with a dying young man. Jay was now completely coherent. With as much determination as his physical strength permitted, Jay demanded that everyone else leave the room. I answered that I would stay with him so that he wouldn't be alone. When he calmly stated that he wanted nothing else done for him, my suspicions were confirmed. When I assured him that I would so inform the doctors, Jay fell silent for a few minutes, only to ask abruptly how much longer he would have to endure this. How I wished I could have ended his suffering! I answered that I didn't know but that I hoped it wouldn't be long. Tears began rolling down my cheeks. Jay brushed his hand across his cheek, as if wiping a tear away, and said "Please don't cry." Then he began to cry. "Sometimes it is not so easy not to cry," was all I could say to him. A few more minutes elapsed, and a dramatic change occurred in Jay. He became peaceful, content, and even happy. As he turned toward me, he winked, smiled, and said, "Thank you." Still crying, I whispered, "You're very welcome, Jay." Moments later he became unconscious, never to recover. As his reflexes diminished, doctors and nurses quietly and gently left the room. Dr. Torpie had arrived, and so we stood, one on either side of the bed, holding his hands until the last reflexes relinquished their control. When this came, we removed the oxygen and covered him. As we left the room, Dr. Torpie said, "Goodbye, Jay."

RT: The room seemed bizarre as a late afternoon sun came through the windows. Nurses and aides came in frequently to document the fleeing blood pressure and pulse. He was comatose, with only his breathing center commanding the dutiful response and rhythm of the lungs to increasing and then decreasing blood levels of carbon dioxide, each cycle becoming shorter and weaker. How many times I had witnessed death and its peace.

He died, and we disconnected the machines, tubes, and switches, sometimes our great friends but now mocking robots to the failure and imperfection of our science. A phone rang in the room. It was for Jay.

REFERENCES

De la Rochefoucauld. Quoted in Wahl, C., 1959. "The Fear of Death." In *The Meaning of Death,* ed. H. Feifel. New York: McGraw-Hill.

Kubler-Ross, E. 1969. *On Death and Dying.* New York: Macmillan.

Norton, J. 1963. "Treatment of the Dying Patient." *Psychoanalytic Study of the Child* 18: 541–60.

Weisman, A. D. 1972. *On Dying and Denying.* New York: Behavioral Publications.

8

The Deadborn Infant: Supportive Care for the Parents

PAULINE M. SEITZ

One of the most striking changes in obstetrical care in the United States during the twentieth century has been the change from home delivery of infants to hospital delivery. With the care of the mother and child transferred from the family to the health-care team in the hospital, many new social customs and medical practices have evolved. The perinatal death rate in the United States has consistently declined, and the parental expectation of having a live, healthy baby has increased accordingly. When tragedy intervenes and the baby dies before or shortly after delivery, the experience is often as foreign and bizarre to the hospital staff as it is to the parents. As one primiparous mother expressed it:

It was all so unreal. When I was in labor I kept thinking—this just can't be happening. I have a good doctor, I had a normal pregnancy, I'm in one of the best hospitals in the country, and I'm having a dead baby. It can't happen—not in real life—babies die in books and movies—this can't be happening to me—not in this day and age.

A rapidly expanding arsenal of prenatal diagnostic tests and tools has made it less common for the medical staff to encounter a stillborn infant. When this does happen, what is traditionally the happiest place in the hospital becomes an acutely uncomfortable place for everyone there. Seitz and Warrick (1974) describe how the staff and parents involved in a perinatal loss cope with the phenomenon. Simultaneously, but at separate and different speeds, each person involved moves through a grief process—not only the parents but also the members of the medical staff and nursing staff, from the time the intrauterine death is diagnosed until discharge from the hospital. Each person integrates the experience differently, according to his degree of involvement. Consequently, the various mechanisms at work may often conflict with one another. Unless the nurse can be aware of where she is and where her patient is, in regard to these mechanisms, there may be an unfortunate break in communication. Grief reactions, to a greater or lesser degree in those involved, can be said to parallel the reactions ascribed to the dying patient by Kubler-Ross (1969).

The mother on a delivery unit with a stillborn infant is committed to a labor that will have no reward. While under tremendous physical and emotional stress, she vacillates through most of the mechanisms of grief work as a means of coping with the loss. Until the actual delivery of the infant, denial persists. The degree to which she needs to maintain denial usually depends on the amount of time she has been aware of the intrauterine demise. If fetal movement has been absent for several days, anticipatory mourning has started, and the mother may be able to say, "It is a relief to finally have it over." One mother expressed this, saying, "It's been dead too long; I want it out so I can live again."

If the death occurs during labor and the mother has been overwhelmed with a battery of people and machines in a desperate search for a different diagnosis, her denial mechanisms are weakened. It is totally incomprehensible that a doctor or nurse could listen to the baby 15 minutes earlier and say all was well, and then listen and say the baby is dead. This is unreal. The situation is stressful and anxiety ridden for everyone. People get angry. The mother is angry that the staff would say such a thing. The staff is angry that they can no longer hear the baby, which means they have failed, through no fault of their own, to save the baby. The father is angry because he has been shoved out of the room, and no one is really telling him what is going on in there. When they finally tell him, he can't believe it, even though he has already concluded that something is very wrong.

A kind of bargaining then follows: "If only I had gone into labor yesterday." Depression spreads throughout the unit. No doctor or nurse wants to go to a delivery room to hear the awful silence of a stillborn birth, but they try to accept it. No one knows what to say to the parents. Everyone is upset. In routine fashion, the mother is sedated. The staff involved in caring for the mother may feel that they are helping the father by deciding that he should leave. Often he is sent off to a waiting room, where he may have to encounter expectant fathers. His only other alternative is to go home and wait helplessly. His wife may interpret this as abandonment. In the midst of the catastrophe of losing an expected infant, further trauma is often added by interfering with or not recognizing the specific individual needs of the bereaved parents.

If the staff involved with the parents are aware of their own feelings and reactions to the situation, they are better able to assist the parents in working through their immediate task of coping with the birth of the infant and the consequent reality of its death. This establishes a foundation for normal grieving responses.

Although a great deal of study has been focused on grief and mourning following the death of adults and children, very little has been done in the area of stillborn infants. A 1970 study done in Chicago by Wolff, Nielson, and Schiller reported that stillbirth is followed by grief but not by depression. None of the 50 women observed in the study had major psychiatric problems as a result of the stillbirth. In a three-year follow-up of 40 of the women, half of them blamed themselves or others for the death, 25 percent attributed it to God's will, and the remaining 25 percent avoided the subject. Yet Cullberg (1972) found that 19 of 56 mothers studied one to two years after the deaths of their neonates had developed severe psychiatric disease. The mortality rate of marriages after a perinatal death, although poorly documented, is well recognized.

Although the literature recommends that parents of stillborn infants be encouraged to ventilate their feelings about the death of the infant and prepare for what feelings they may encounter at home, virtually no mention is made of whether or not the parents should be given the option of seeing the baby. In many hospitals parents are actively discouraged from seeing the baby because it will be "too upsetting," "make them hysterical," or "make it all much worse." There are no data in the literature to support this viewpoint as a standard. This attitude may reflect the feelings of the staff and not the parents. Very often the option of seeing the baby is not even raised to the parents. If it is, it is often presented with obvious ambivalence on the part of the staff: "You don't want to see the baby, do you?" This is not offering the parents a choice; it is presenting them with a challenge. While still under sedation, many women will follow the staff's lead. It is only later that the mother may begin to think, "What was it that they didn't want me to see?"

The nurse must be aware that some parents can cope better with grief when the reality of seeing and touching the baby has been enacted. Engel (1964) states:

The need to touch the dying or dead person is of overwhelming importance to some and will not be requested by those for whom it will be disturbing. Rituals provide some of the most important external supports for the grief-stricken and are often essential to their ability to tolerate the first period of intense distress.

When a stillborn infant was delivered at home, the family was responsible for and involved in the arrangements surrounding the burial of the child. In the hospital setting, the baby is often quickly removed to the morgue. For some parents this can create intolerable tension. They must know what their child was like to assimilate the loss. The sex and the weight of the baby are only statistics. The parents need more personalized information to make their stillborn an individual, not a thing.

The nurse can play an invaluable role in helping the parents at this time. One mother, recalling her feelings as she woke up on the delivery table after delivering a deadborn, said: "For the first time in my life, I understand the phrase 'dead silence.'" It is often up to the nurse, who is alone with the mother, to break the silence. Her perception of the baby is the first and, therefore, the most important one the mother will receive. The nurse determines whether it was "a boy, seven pounds," or "a son, seven pounds, with brown hair, blue eyes, big feet and long fingernails." The attention to details about the baby is important, for it conveys care and concern for the infant. This is a signal to the mother that she did not deliver a creature so repulsive no one wanted to look at it.

The parents should be asked individually and separately what their feelings are about seeing the baby. This allows them to express themselves in an unbiased atmosphere. It has been the experience of this author that parents who will find the experience of seeing the infant distressful do not hesitate to say so. Parents who are ambivalent will ask the nurse what she thinks they should do. The nurse should explain that it is a very individualized decision and one that she cannot make for them. She can only support their needs. The nurse can then explain what the baby looks like, and if the infant is macerated or deformed, she should carefully describe its appearance.

The following case presentation consists of excerpts from a process recording by this author. The patient, Mrs. S., was a 30-year-old married primipara who, despite an uncomplicated pregnancy, delivered a deadborn infant at term. Five days before delivery, when the patient went to see her physician after a 24-hour absence of fetal movement, the diagnosis of intrauterine demise was made. Since the cervix was unsuitable for induction of labor, her physician carefully explained what had happened and why he could not admit her for induction at that time. He maintained close contact with Mrs. S. until she arrived at the hospital in active labor. At that time she was placed under sedation. The author met her on the delivery unit 40 minutes after she had been sedated. Mrs. S. was alert and responsive with no visible affective response to the sedation. She was doing her La Maze breathing techniques with her husband.

When the husband left the room to talk with the doctor, the author introduced the subject of seeing the baby.

NURSE: Have you thought about whether or not you would like to see the baby?

MRS. S.: I have been. I don't know what to think. I want to see the baby but not if it will make it worse. I mean if there is something really wrong. The baby's been dead so long, that must change things—I don't know what to do.

NURSE: It's always a difficult question, and there is no perfect answer. I can tell you what the baby will look like. When the circulation stops and the baby dies—for whatever reason—changes start to take place. The skin will be red and peeling—like a very bad sunburn. The bones in the head tend to mold more and they become very soft. The red peeling skin and softness of the head can be a severe shock when you have never seen it before. The staff can see past that to what is normal about your baby. It may be too disconcerting and therefore distressful for you to see past it. Think about what you would like to do. When the baby is born, I will tell you what I see and we can talk about it then. Whatever you want to do is the right thing.

In the delivery room, Mrs. S. was given inhalation analgesia. She pushed the head halfway out and was given general anesthesia. A deadborn girl was delivered. Marked constriction of the cord was noted at the umbilicus and near the insertion of the placenta. When Mrs. S. woke up, her doctor had gone to talk to her husband.

NURSE: It's all right to wake up now. It's all over.

MRS. S.: (reaching for her abdomen and touching it) Is it really over? I don't remember having the baby. I was pushing. I remember up till then.

NURSE: It's a little girl—perfectly formed. There was a problem with her umbilical cord. It was twisted and it cut off her circulation. She is a normal baby with fuzzy brown hair.

MRS. S.: She doesn't have three eyes or no legs?

NURSE: No, she is a normal baby, but her skin is red and peeling. Think about whether or not you want to see her.

MRS. S.: I do want to see her.

NURSE: I will show her to you.

MRS. S.: May I see her now?

NURSE: Let's wait until your husband is here. Maybe he would like to see her.

MRS. S.: I don't know if he wants to.

NURSE: We'll ask him.

When Mr. S. arrived, his wife told him she wanted to see the baby.

MR. S.: There is no need for you to see that baby. Dr. F. has told us it was a normal girl and they will do an autopsy. It was a defective cord and there is no need to see her.

The nurse left the room without comment.

Mr. S. stayed with the patient for about half an hour. When he left the unit, the following conversation took place with his wife:

MRS. S.: May I see my baby now? My husband doesn't want to see her, but I've been thinking about it and I have to see her. What do you think? Will it be bad for me to see her?

NURSE: I don't know. It would be bad for you to spend the rest of your life wondering about it. You have to do whatever feels most comfortable for you. For some people, seeing the baby is too disturbing. For others, it is the only way they can accept that it really happened. I don't want you to spend the rest of your life thinking there was anything we tried to hide from you because your doctor, your husband, or I thought it would hurt too much to tell you. The baby will not look pale and white. Her skin is very red and peeling like a bad sunburn. Her head is very molded and soft.

The baby was carried into the room wrapped in a blanket. As many personal touches as possible in showing the baby should be used—a pink or blue blanket, the regulation baby bracelet. Holding the baby shows that the nurse is not afraid to touch the child. It recognizes that this infant is someone the mother carried inside her.

MRS. S.:   The poor little thing.

NURSE: It didn't hurt her. It only hurts us. She would have been a beautiful daughter. Who has the cleft chin in your family?

MRS. S.:   You're kidding! My husband does—does she really have one?

Mrs. S. then examined the baby from head to toe. She was particularly interested in seeing exactly where the cord was twisted and constricted. We then discussed how this was an apparently normal baby who, despite the very best of care, had a tragic but unpreventable accident. It was no one's fault.

Ten minutes later, after the baby had been carried out:

MRS. S.:   This may sound funny, but it was a relief to see her. It really is over now. I know she was a normal baby. I'm going to have another one as soon as I can. I'm not going to let this stop me. . . . It was right for me to see her.

NURSE: Everyone's protective mechanisms are different. Your husband couldn't see her and he shouldn't have. He seems to be coping by intellectualizing the experience—a cause and an effect. It's very different for a mother though. You were the only one who really knew the baby. You were the one who first felt her move and stop moving. It's much harder for you to accept her death. There was no way you could believe she was really dead until it happened. You have to believe we were all wrong or you would have gone crazy.

MRS. S.:   It's so true—but now it is over.

After Mrs. S. was brought downstairs to her room, the following conversation took place with her husband:

NURSE: Your wife wanted to see the baby after you left. I brought the baby to her. It seemed to comfort her. I had a "gut feeling" it was right for her. I think it would have been wrong for you. I don't want you to think we were sneaking around behind your back. There aren't any rules when this happens—only feelings. It's my job to take care of both of you.

MR. S.:   That's okay. It's not a problem. Really, it's not a problem. Thank you for everything you've done.

The nurse who has been with the parents during labor and delivery should maintain close contact with them while the mother is in the hospital. This nurse can provide, discuss, and clarify details about the infant and the labor and delivery experience because she is one of the few people who had contact with the baby. Her information can be crucial in the mother's future attitude toward pregnancy and delivery. Mourning is enabled on the basis of reality and fact, not on fantasy. A pregnancy that terminates with a deadborn infant produces a tremendous sense of failure in parental role identity. By seeking the parents out and allowing them to ventilate their feelings, the labor nurse can help restore some self-esteem. These parents are often left in an aura of sympathetic isolation by staff members. The staff's rationale is, "Don't disturb them in their grief." The parents' interpretation of this may be, "They don't care very much."

The nurse can facilitate communication between the

parents and staff by explaining why this isolation occurs. No one knows what to say, and so often nothing is said. Sometimes platitudes, such as "Next time you'll have a healthy baby and forget all about this," are offered by well-intentioned staff members. At this time, the present loss—and not their future children—is the primary concern of the parents.

Before they leave the hospital, the parents should be prepared for what they may encounter at home. If delivery of a deadborn infant is an increasingly less common experience in the hospital setting, it is even more so in the community of family and friends. The parents will encounter people who say too little or people who ask too much about the baby. Within the structure of their marriage it is an extremely stressful time for the parents. One parent may be eager to talk about the baby at a time when the other needs silence. By maintaining contact with parents, the nurse may help them understand the mechanisms they are using to cope with their grief. Her continued interest after the mother's discharge from the hospital can help the parents assimilate the loss of the infant into their family life.

REFERENCES

Cullberg, J. 1972. "Mental Reactions of Women to Perinatal Death." In *Psychosomatic Medicine in Obstetrics and Gynecology,* ed. N. Morris. New York : S. Karger.

Engel, G. 1964. "Grief and Grieving." *The American Journal of Nursing* 64, No. 9 (September):93–98.

Kubler-Ross, E. 1969. *On Death and Dying.* New York: Macmillan.

Seitz, P. and L. Warrick. 1974. "Perinatal Death: The Grieving Mother." *The American Journal of Nursing* 74, No. 11 (November):2028–33.

Wolff, J. R., P. E. Neilson, and P. Schiller. 1970. "The Emotional Reaction to a Stillbirth." *American Journal of Obstetrics and Gynecology* 108 (September 1):73–77.

9

Therapeutic Intervention with the Bereaved

JAY ROGERS
and
M. L. S. VACHON

At present, it would seem that nursing interest and involvement in thanatology have been concentrated mainly in responding to the needs of gravely ill and dying patients and their families. Nurses, by the very nature of their personal caring roles, have been the professionals on the spot when dying occurs in institutional settings. However, attention should be focused on the ways in which nursing skills can be used and expanded to help the survivors of death—the bereaved.

The physical, emotional, and social aftereffects of the stress of bereavement, with particular reference to widows and widowers, are well documented, and more in-depth research is in process. The impact of bereavement has been viewed as an illness (Peretz, 1970), as a crisis (Maddison and Viola, 1968; Raphael, 1971), and as a psychosocial transition (Parkes, 1970). Other authors have studied the effects of bereavement by using such indicators as physical and mental illness, and death, including suicide (Glaser and Strauss, 1972; Kraus and Lilienfeld, 1959; Maddison, 1971; Parkes, 1964, 1965). It is now known that the incidence of somatic and emotional problems and mortality rates in the bereaved are much higher than in the normal population.

Surely, the role of the nurse, however concretely defined, falls within the parameters of the above-mentioned researched areas. There have, however, been problems, both specific to nursing and general to all of the health professions, that have led to the present situation wherein the widowed are often not offered help pertinent to the stress of bereavement.

For years, nurses have been encouraged to take into account the environment, the family, and various social and emotional needs when making a care plan for a patient. However, death increasingly takes place in institutions rather than at home, and institutions rarely have mechanisms whereby the staff can continue to reach out to families after death occurs. When the patient dies, the family disappears; and the nurses transfer their attentions to new patients. Glaser and Strauss (1972) discuss this as they look at the impact of social loss on nurses. They also point out that the family can be forgotten even before death occurs, in instances such as a lingering illness or a comatose state where visits taper off.

One institution that has developed mechanisms to enable staff to reach out to families of terminally ill patients and to arrange for help after death occurs is St. Christopher's Hospice in England. The nurses have been very much involved in carrying out this responsibility (Twycross, 1975). There are a few examples in other parts of the world where this approach is being considered or tested currently, but in Canada no such organized programs are known to us, although one of the authors is involved in preliminary work in this area in a cancer hospital.

Few instances are known of nurses working in community settings and consciously setting up mechanisms or programs to offer counseling specific to acute grief and bereavement. An important contribution to preventive medicine could be made by public health nurses, nurse practitioners, psychiatric nurses, industrial nurses, and others if they were helped to feel competent to give service in this area. Indeed, it is amazing that more emphasis is not placed on continued care for the bereaved at all levels of nursing education and in-service programs.

A strong educational beginning has been made in some parts of the United States and Canada (Wagner, 1972; Watson, 1972), but we are still far from the optimum goal of having thanatology included as a nursing prerequisite. It would seem also that, insofar as the stresses of bereavement are concerned, there are few examples for nurses to follow if they wish to apply in practice whatever theoretical knowledge they have been taught.

Many professionals feel inadequate in grief counseling. It is difficult enough to shoulder the responsibility of dealing with the emotional needs of the dying, who are directly involved as recipients of professional attention. The bereaved, however, are in the community; and it is still a widely held assumption (or rationalization) that they will require only the technical services of doctors and nurses and that they will request these services as they need them (Dobrof, 1972). Health professionals are busy people and can mask their feelings of inadequacy in terms of time pressures and their subsequent preference for giving concrete treatment or advice rather than emotional support over a period of indeterminate length. Thus doctors may medicate, clergymen may urge prayer and faith, and social agency workers may attempt to identify legal, financial, vocational problems, and so forth. Nurses frequently direct people to these professionals while also advocating support of the family.

Families and friends gather round for a while, offering much support and advice. Then they tend to take up their own lives again or fall away because the grieving process fills them with uncomfortable feelings and perhaps out of general frustration because the bereaved person is not responding so quickly as expected. Thus "the buck" continues to be "passed," and nobody takes continuing responsibility for a service that is really required.

The following case history is only one illustration of how nursing skills can be used in counseling the bereaved. The authors have been researching the stresses of bereavement and developing a program of intervention for the newly bereaved.* In addition their clinical responsibilities include responding to requests for individual bereavement counseling.

Mrs. F. is a 63-year-old woman whose husband died suddenly of a massive coronary 1½ years ago. He had been a successful businessman, and was a warm, capable person, well liked by everyone. Mrs. F. had been very dependent upon him and had always had difficulty making decisions. For years she had suffered from mild phobias, had had several episodes of psychosomatic symptomatology, and was seen by friends and family as rather self-concerned, nagging, and complaining. Her husband drank moderately to cope with her. Her family physician, a close friend of the husband, tolerated her frequent visits and gave her token medication when she complained. In the last five years of her husband's life, her three children left home, one by one, to marry, and her aged father, who lived with the family, died.

After her husband's death, she deteriorated emotionally. Her children and her social network had related to her husband rather than to her. An entire support structure had disappeared, and her overwhelming dependency needs were unmet. Those who reached out to her found that she latched onto them completely, and so they either fell away or attempted to give her large amounts of conflicting advice. Her children were unwilling to consider having her move in with them, even though this is what she was requesting. They were extremely frustrated by their mother's behavior and were unaware of the dynamics involved. The doctor became less tolerant and suggested she admit herself to a private sanitorium, a suggesion she resisted. She became increasingly agitated and depressed and began to lose weight. Finally, she decided to go to the emergency department of the Clarke Institute and en route became involved in a car accident that resulted in severe facial contusions and lacerations.

It was decided that it would be preferable to avoid starting her on a "patient career" if at all possible, and she was referred to our service as a problem surrounding adjustment to widowhood. For two months, she has been seen regularly on an outpatient basis and has made a steady improvement. The treatment approach has been to use both the knowledge of the dynamics of bereavement and the

* Research supported by Ontario Ministry of Health Demonstration Model Grant No. DM 158.

dynamics of Mrs. F.'s premorbid personality and to help her explore her feelings in a positive, supportive manner. Her family and her physician were involved from the outset. Their new understanding of the situation and their relief that professional support is available have enabled them to adjust their expectations and to offer Mrs. F. more appropriate help.

In addition to counseling the newly bereaved, nurses can also provide support for those anticipating bereavement. It is hoped that such counseling will decrease some of the stress that occurs in the newly bereaved.

Mrs. B. is a 35-year-old mother of two children who was referred to one of the authors because of difficulty in adjusting to the impending death of her husband. The nursing staff on the unit where he was hospitalized for radiation therapy complained that Mrs. B. was extremely angry because she felt her husband's brain tumor should have been diagnosed sooner than it was. She seemed incapacitated by her anger, and this was causing hospital personnel, as well as family and friends, to reject her, a fact that added more fuel to her anger.

For the first three therapy sessions Mrs. B. did little questioning other than angrily reviewing her husband's symptoms and questioning why he was not diagnosed earlier. Her hostility toward the doctors was extremely marked because she felt they had missed the diagnosis and then operated too late and made her husband a "vegetable" whom they were sending now to a chronic care hospital so that they would not have to see "their mistake."

She was accompanied to the first three sessions by family members, and the therapist assumed that this was because of some resistance and the need to feel family support. For the fourth session she came alone, and her anger dissolved into the tears of depression as she began to grieve for the loss of the husband she had known. Watching this meticulous man regress and become incontinent, she began to face the fact that he was dying. She stated that she came to see the therapist because the therapist was the only person who would talk about the fact that her husband was indeed dying. Doctors evaded her, and family members tried to reassure her that her husband would soon be well. She felt completely alone as she tried to accept the reality of his death and found it easier to maintain her hostility than to face her depression.

As she began to grieve, Mrs. B.'s anger decreased considerably, but she still felt her husband had been misdiagnosed, and she wanted to do something about it. She was encouraged in this because it was felt that this could decrease the impotence she felt and help her to mobilize her resources. She decided to write to the Medical Director of the hospital and was accompanied by the therapist to the ensuing interview. This gave her the satisfaction of feeling that, although her husband would die, his death and the suffering it caused would not go unnoticed.

After two months in therapy Mrs. B. is now able to face her husband's impending death and to talk openly about this with her children. Her anger has decreased considerably, but she remains sufficiently aggressive to ensure that her husband receives good care while in the chronic care facility.

These two anecdotes reveal some of the ways in which nurses can facilitate the work of bereavement. Although neither case can be considered a model instance of bereavement, it is hoped that they show some of the problems faced by the bereaved and those anticipating bereavement. Additionally, they reveal that the nurse can have a role in bereavement counseling.

Along with the responsibilities associated with their research project and their clinical work with the bereaved, the authors are becoming increasingly involved in the education of nurses, other disciplines, and lay groups. Not only is it important to increase awareness and knowledge within the nursing profession, but also nursing has "the obligation to take an active role in the education of the general public" (Britten, 1972).

To contribute effectively in this area of preventive medicine, nurses must be prepared to enlarge upon the traditionally defined scope of their roles and accept more responsibility while at the same time advocating a multidisciplinary approach (Benoliel, 1972). The rewards of this sort of commitment for the nurse who is willing to take these steps are many—not only in personal, clinical satisfaction but also in the "ripple effect" that ensues as awareness levels in the community are raised and additional counseling services and "a more imaginative use of traditional practices" (Jackson, 1972) are achieved.

REFERENCES

Benoliel, J. Q. 1972. "Nursing Care for the Terminal Patient: A Psychosocial Approach." In *Psychosocial Aspects of Terminal Care,* ed. B. Schoenberg et al., pp. 145–161, New York: Columbia University Press.

Britten, M. 1972. "Nursing Workshop." In *Psychosocial Aspects of Terminal Care,* ed. B. Schoenberg et al. New York: Columbia University Press.

Bunch, J. 1972. "Recent Bereavement in Relation to Suicide." *Journal of Psychosomatic Research* 16:361.

Dobrof, R. 1972. "Community Resources and the Care of the Terminally Ill and Their Families." In *Psychosocial Aspects of Terminal Care,* ed. B. Schoenberg et al. pp. 290–306, New York: Columbia University Press.

Glaser, A. G. and A. L. Strauss. 1972. "The Social Loss a Dying Patient." In *The Dying Patient: A Nursing Perspective,* ed. M. H. Browning and E. P. Lewis. New York: The American Journal of Nursing Company.

Jackson, E. N. 1972. "The Importance of Understanding Grief." In *Religion and Bereavement,* ed. A. H. Kutscher and L. G. Kutscher. New York: Health Sciences Publishing Corporation.

Kraus, A. S. and A. M. Lilienfeld. 1959. "Some Epidemiological Aspects of the High Mortality Rate in the Young Widowed Group." *Journal of Chronic Diseases* 10:207.

Maddison, D. 1971. "The Sting of Death." Paper presented at St. Michael's Hospital, Toronto (December).

Maddison, D. and A. Viola. 1968. "The Health of Widows in the Year Following Bereavement." *Journal of Psychosomatic Research* 12:297.

Parkes, C. M. 1964. "Effects of Bereavement on Physical and Mental Health: A Study of the Medical Records of Widows." *British Medical Journal* 2:274.

———— 1965. "Bereavement and Mental Illness: Part I, A Clinical Study of the Grief of Bereaved Psychiatric Patients." *British Journal of Medical Psychology* 38:1.

———— 1970. "Psychosocial Transitions: A Field for Study." *Social Sciences and Medicine* 5:101.

Peretz, D. 1970. "Reaction to Loss." In *Loss and Grief: Psychological Man-*

agement in Medical Practice, ed. B. Schoenberg et al., pp. 20–35. New York: Columbia University Press.

Raphael, B. 1971. "Crisis Intervention: Theoretical and Methodological Considerations." *Australian–New Zealand Journal of Psychiatry* 5:183.

Twycross, R. 1976. "Acute Grief: A Physician's Viewpoint." In *Acute Grief and the Funeral,* ed. V. R. Pine et al. Springfield, Illinois: Charles C Thomas.

Wagner, B. M. 1972. "Teaching Students to Work with the Dying," In *The Dying Patient: A Nursing Perspective,* ed. M. H. Browning and E. P. Lewis. New York: The American Journal of Nursing Company.

Watson, M. J. 1972. "Death—A Necessary Concern for Nurses." In *The Dying Patient: A Nursing Perspective,* ed. M. H. Browning and E. P. Lewis. New York: The American Journal of Nursing Company.

Coping
Problems of
Professionals~~~~~~~~~~~~~~~~~~~~~

PART TWO

10

Working Through Feelings Around Death

JUNE S. LOWENBERG

In areas related to death and dying, perhaps more than in any others involving health personnel, theoretical constructs are not enough to help a person function clinically. A nurse with deep knowledge and skills in relation to communication, the grief process, and how people cope with impending and actual death may not be able to use research findings until she can handle her emotional reactions to the many painful experiences she will confront in working with people facing death.

Nurses use so much energy to handle their own feelings that, as a result, they may not be able to recognize or deal with the patient's needs. Because of the highly charged emotional impact of our concerns with death, it becomes difficult to prevent our feelings and needs from interfering with those of the patient. Beyond the obvious examples where the nurse's needs result in physical avoidance of a patient or emotional distancing from him, actions based on a nurse's assumptions often leave patients' needs unmet.

For example, a nurse may decide a terminally ill patient needs peaceful surroundings, because a "good death," to her, is tranquil. For one patient, providing a serene environment may be therapeutic; however, another person might view serenity as "predeath" at a time when he is struggling to maintain optimal stimulation during the time remaining in his life. Or the nurse may project her fear of pain onto the patient. Pain may be the greatest fear of many in relation to dying, and yet some people may view pain as evidence of life. These examples are oversimplifications and ignore the complexity of variables in problems of sensory stimulation and pain, but they remind us of how easily we impute our perceptions and needs to patients.

Each nurse is likely to continue to meet her own needs and assess the patient's needs in relation to her own until she at least partially works through her feelings about dying and death. As long as a patient's question, "Am I going to die?" or his request, "Please, help me to die," evokes an overwhelming emotional reaction, the nurse probably will not be able to remain in the situation, much less identify and attempt to meet the person's needs. Working through feelings about death may be the most important process necessary to improve nursing care in this area, and it is the most difficult. To develop a personal philosophy of life and death, one must think about and expose oneself to many painful experiences.

First, I need to clarify my assumption that, in stressing the need for developing a philosophy, I do not advocate that such a viewpoint be imposed on others. Only if the nurse is aware of her feelings and beliefs can she see beyond them to the other person's experience. Often her beliefs about an afterlife, for example, differ significantly from the patient's; she needs to be aware of her own beliefs and reactions to keep them from interfering with her ability to provide support for the patient within his own philosophical framework.

Developing a thoughtful philosophy of life and death presents a monumental and continuing challenge. For me it remains easier to discuss this than to go through the process itself. Introspection is probably the keystone to initiating this process. Reading and discussions with others about death provide further avenues for developing one's views and working through one's feelings. Along with this, each nurse must also formulate her philosophy of nursing and professionalism to work effectively in these areas.

Introspection in this area is extremely painful. First, each nurse can examine her thoughts and feelings about death in general. Most of us experience unpleasant reactions of fear or anxiety or revulsion when we begin to think about death. These reactions are often compelling enough to make us feel as though something must be wrong with us. It is important to remember continually how normal these feelings are. Recognizing how common these reactions are sometimes makes them a little easier to live with.

What does she see as the meaning of life and death? Does she live for pleasure and enjoyment of the moment, for improving the welfare of others, or for certain types of achievement? Does she conceptualize death as a void, a loss of everything meaningful; as a transition to another state; or as the completion of a cyclic pattern? What constitutes dying a "good death" to her? And at what point does she define a person as "dead"?

Examining feelings around death in general evokes memories of previous experiences with death, both professional and personal, and these open up new areas for exploration. Often these previous experiences, especially if they occurred when the person was vulnerable, color all further reactions to situations involving dying or grief.

The nursing student's initial contact with a dying person is often so overwhelming that it prevents her from involving herself with similar experiences. A young and inexperienced student may be left to cope with the complex problems associated with a dying patient because the clinical and teaching staff are unable to handle their own reactions to the situation (Quint, 1967). The student then feels abandoned and isolated, while experiencing overwhelming feelings of helplessness; these feelings persist and interfere as she approaches similar situations in the future. Confronting these memories of deaths, as well as those that appeared to be more peaceful or beautiful, can help her work out some of her unresolved feelings about this kind of experience.

Examining her feelings around personal experience with death can also help. Trying to think of the first time she became aware of death and how she felt can clarify some of her present reactions. Each time she experiences a death, these feelings arise, and often grief still unresolved from these earlier contacts prevents her from dealing with the current situation.

As she thinks through her feelings about previous encounters with dying and death, feelings about her own potential death arise. Although this may be the most painful part of introspection, unless she starts becoming aware of these feelings, she cannot be comfortable with allowing others to explore their feelings about their impending death. Has she made any preparations for her eventual death in terms of life insurance, wills, and funeral arrangements? How and when does she envision her own death will occur?

The nurse who wants to deal more effectively with her feelings about death must also explore her feelings about strong emotions, such as anger and sorrow. Grief requires an active expression of both angry and sad feelings. Typically, in our society, these feelings should be kept under control with minimal outward expression. If the nurse reacts negatively to the expression of strong feelings, it will be extremely difficult for her to assist people facing death. Not only will she have to deal with their hostility and grief, she may often be experiencing these emotions herself. Can she help someone express his sorrow if she believes that outward display of such emotion is a sign of weakness or even immorality? Can she assist a person who is wailing or crying loudly if she feels grief should be expressed only in private? And are those feelings so horrible that she will not allow herself to recognize them when she experiences them personally?

The nurse must also confront her feelings about working directly with people who are dying or dead. How does she react when she thinks of caring for terminal patients? Is she more comfortable in a role where she has numerous technical responsibilities that allow her to minimize direct patient interaction, avoiding listening to and sharing the struggles of a person facing his own death? How does she react when she imagines touching a dead body or watching a family caress and talk to a person who has just died?

Moving beyond introspection, the nurse can further develop her philosophy through reading about life and death. The work of individuals facing death, their own or that of someone close, can be especially helpful to the nurse who has had relatively slight personal experiences with death (Agee, 1963; Alsop, 1974; de Beauvoir, 1966; Gunther, 1949; Wertenbaker, 1957). Solzhenitsyn's *The Cancer Ward* (1969) provided me with more powerful insights into the experiences surrounding death than any professional work.

In the last decade the body of professional literature dealing with death and grief has been expanding. Feifel's interdisciplinary anthology *The Meaning of Death* (1959) remains a landmark, as does Fulton's *Death and Identity* (1965). The perspectives available through the fields of philosophy (Choron, 1963), sociology (Glaser and Strauss, 1965, 1968; Sudnow, 1967), psychology (Kastenbaum and Aisenberg, 1972), psychiatry (Kubler-Ross, 1969; Schoenberg et al., 1970; Weisman, 1972), and theology (Fletcher, 1973; Grollman, 1967; Neale, 1973; Weber, 1973) raise varied issues for incorporation into one's professional and personal philosophy of death. The nursing literature has also increasingly reflected the concerns arising from recognizing the complexities of the problems posed by death, loss, and grief (*American Journal of Nursing*, 1972; Quint, 1967). The length of the most recent bibliography of death, grief, and bereavement compiled by Fulton (1973) for the Center for Death Education and Research attests to the publication explosion in thanatology. The parallel explosion of audiovisual materials relating to death provides still further resources for exploring these perspectives. A workshop on terminal illness for health professionals in death education at the University of Washington in 1974 offered 39 films for viewing, along with a multitude of videotapes and audiotapes. A few examples include "How Could I Not Be Among You?," "The Day Grandpa Died," "Widow," "You See—I've Had a Life," "Dead Man," and "Until I Die."

Discussions with other professionals provide one of the most promising avenues to developing one's philosophy of life and death. Sharing experiences and feelings with nurses can broaden one's perspective, while providing mutual support. Individual and group discussions with other health professionals and the clergy can also raise and explore the numerous issues that arise around death.

Theologians can provide information about belief systems and the formalized rituals of dying of the various religions. Psychiatrists and psychologists can often bring supportive input to a nurse or group of nurses trying to work through their feelings around dying or around a particular death. (A clinical specialist or mental health consultant should assume a similar role within nursing.)

Sharing information and support in direct interaction and collaboration with physicians may be the most important approach in attempts to improve the care of the dying and their families (actually, interdisciplinary education in this area may be necessary for this teamwork to emerge). Both the nurse and the physician, as functioning members of American society, bring the attitudes and values of the larger society in relation to death into their work. Relegating death to institutional settings, such as the hospital and extended care facilities, may protect society as a whole; however, it cannot protect those entrusted with the care of the people dying within those settings.

Added to this strain is the cure orientation the nurse and physician share as members of the health team. If the team's primary shared goal involves "curing" people and "saving lives" (many physicians would include "preventing death" in these goals), each death of a patient serves as a symbol of failure.

Dr. M., a young pediatric intern, was in charge of an adolescent dying of Hodgkins disease. His first patient death had occurred two weeks earlier, also a young adolescent. He was able to verbalize to me his feelings that he was a failure as a physician and, with much emotion, he talked of his consideration of leaving medicine after giving so much time to his education.

The nurse has a slight advantage over the physician in this area, since her unique contribution to medicine is seen as "care" rather than "cure." Whether the goal of "care" is conceived of as maintaining behavioral equilibrium, helping the patient adapt to the stresses accompanying disease or treatment, or reducing stress and promoting comfort, these goals are clearly differentiated from those of helping the patient achieve optimal health or saving his life. Once a patient is defined as dying, the nurse can concentrate her efforts on helping the person cope with the overwhelming stresses affecting him and on providing emotional and physical comfort. The doctor does not view this as his area of expertise and, because of the increased burden his cure orientation places on him, I believe the nurse may have to take the responsibility for providing support to the physician in this area.

I asked Dr. M. what his goals were in working with his patient, and he immediately replied to "save" him. Together we discussed whether that was realistic in this instance; why should a young and still inexperienced doctor expect himself to do what the top specialists in the country had been unable to accomplish? We explored together what goals might be more reasonable at this point. When Dr. M. felt that comfort might be more appropriate, I pointed out that intervention in this area was my primary responsibility, although I needed support from him in carrying this out. I also tried to help him view his sensitivity toward this patient as one of his strengths, indicating his potential within medicine.

This view of nurse–physician collaboration departs from the tradition of nurses as the physician's handmaidens. If a physician said a patient was not to be told the diagnosis or prognosis, a nurse would say, "What can I do?"—even if it were obvious to her, from the patient's comments, that he was fully aware of his impending death and had a strong need to share his fears.

The nurse is often the person with the most knowledge about the patient and family, their concerns and fears, and their attempts to cope with these problems. This information must be shared, just as the nurse needs to know the patient's medical status. As in the example of the young intern, the nurse should become both accountable and responsible for the patient's "care." Traditionally, again, this has not happened (Strauss and Quint, 1964). Especially in cases that involved dying, with the intense involvement and guilt that are present, I believe doctors should share the decision-making with the nurses.

Steven, a 16-year-old boy, in the advanced stages of Hodgkins disease, had been increasingly speaking of death and his wish to die during the week preceding his death. He told me and other staff members that, if we wouldn't let him die, he would have to find a way himself. After this statement, he refused food, saying it would only make things "last longer." He repeatedly asked me to help him by getting him some poison so that he could end his life faster (he also asked one of the doctors). He cried frequently, verbalizing his pain and helplessness and his inability to "take it" any more. During this period many life-prolonging measures were being used, including repeated thoracenteses. Morphine was being withheld because of the danger of further impairing respiration.

After much thought and soul-searching about what I perceived as Steven's needs versus my own, I decided I was negating my responsibility. I then approached the head of the service, telling about Steve's reactions and saying that I felt that we were now meeting our own needs rather than his. The physician told me that I did not need to share in the decision-making around stopping some of the prolonging measures and beginning morphine. It was very tempting to leave then, but I felt I had to remain and participate in the decision, which was as much my responsibility as theirs (Lowenberg, 1970).

Assuming this type of relationship with the physician involves numerous risks for the nurse. She must acknowledge her accountability to herself and to physicians (neither one may view this very favorably!). She must be able to back up her decisions with her reasoning and sound theoretical data. And she must be prepared for the consequences of threatening physicians who view their role as that of the unquestioned authority in all aspects of patient care. For me, the most difficult part was exposing myself to the painful burden of participating in similar decisions. The nurse must first have carefully thought out her feelings in terms of her values. Where does she place her highest priority: on the physician's approval? on the estimation of her superior or peers in the nursing hierarchy? on her responsibility to her patient?

A nurse's philosophy of nursing affects her interactions with fatally ill patients as much as her philosophy of life and death. Each nurse must decide what nursing encompasses and the degree to which it is oriented toward curative or care goals. If nursing aims primarily to promote comfort and alleviate suffering, how can we justify communicating with patients around areas that may evoke crying and obvious emotional distress? How do we balance our goals of promoting growth and providing comfort, when meaningful growth is painful? I know that there are no simple answers for any of us.

I believe another area of nursing philosophy is extremely important for any nurse working with the dying. What are her beliefs about respect for others and dignity? Numerous writings discuss the importance of providing "dignity" to the dying patient, but what is her definition of dignity? And how does a nurse provide it? One component is respect for the person's individual, cultural, and religious values and active use of this value system as a base in all interactions with the patient.

Another component of respect and dignity relates to beliefs about trust and honesty versus pretense in nurse—patient relationships. How much should the patient be told, and is there justification for lying? Does the patient have a right to know his disease condition and prognosis? If so, who should tell him and how? If a patient is not told his prognosis, does that deprive him of knowledge that might alter the decisions he makes before his death? Does pretense dehumanize a patient? Each nurse must have at least partially resolved these questions before she can feel comfortable in allowing a patient to share his concerns with her.

What kind of contracts do physicians and nurses establish with their patients? In the hospital we strip patients of their rights and choices around even such simple areas as dressing and eating. What about the way they die? How much control or choice should a patient or his family have? One patient, for example, may want every possible measure taken to prolong his life, or it may be very important to his family that this take place. Another patient may want to die. Do we intervene similarly in both cases? As we intervene, how can we be sure that we are using judgment based on the patient's needs rather than our own? This introduces still broader questions, not only in relation to euthanasia, but in relation to suicide (one could even ask whether nurses and doctors have a right to prevent suicide).

Often, whatever the patient has been told by his physician, he directs questions at the nurse, such as "Am I going to die?" Actually the patient may not be asking for an answer. He may be asking whether the disease he has is fatal or whether he is in the process of dying now. Or he may be seeking reassurance that he is not dying. It is also likely that he knows that he is dying, but that he is attempting to find out whether the nurse will be honest with him or whether she is willing to listen as he talks about his concerns. Usually, these other concerns and questions are what he wishes to discuss. Listening becomes much more important than providing "answers." As Benoliel (1970) writes:

Any time that a patient spontaneously introduces the topic of his dying, whether by a question or by a statement, he is telling you that he desperately needs to establish communication with another human being and that he needs help in coping with what is happening to him.

Pulling up a chair offers one way to communicate one's willingness to listen, and many of the most effective ways to demonstrate concern involve nonverbal communication and touch.

The issue of professionalism arises from one's philosophy of nursing. Each nurse must develop her beliefs about what constitutes professional action as a helping person. Perhaps the major issues in this area revolve around involvement with patients and families. Should a nurse maintain a "professional" barrier or distance when relating to a patient, or should she attempt to know the patient as a person, removing many of these barriers? Does the nurse empathize or sympathize with patients she cares for? Should the nurse care about the patient as a person?

The nurse often protects herself by minimizing her involvement with patients and families. Jourard (1971, p. 781) graphically describes the bedside manner as:

. . . character armor . . . acquired (by a nurse) as a means of coping with the anxieties engendered by repeated encounters with suffering, demanding patients. . . . If the "armor" is effective, it permits the nurse to go about her duties unaffected by any disturbing feelings of pity, anger, inadequacy, or insecurity.

Professional distance protects the nurse from these threatening feelings in herself in response to a patient's behavior. If she has allowed herself to care deeply for a dying patient, his death may represent a personal loss to her; in contrast, if she remains detached, his death cannot "get to her." Does this protection from pain allow her to grow as a human being? If she does not allow herself to be aware of her grief or anger or helplessness, can she work through these feelings?

Initially, a nurse may have become involved with her patients and been exposed to many such disturbing experiences without receiving support within or outside the work setting. No matter how idealistic the intent, I believe a person can continue to expose herself without support only for a limited period before she begins to raise defenses to insulate herself.

The consequences for the patient of nursing care that is technically competent but performed at an emotional distance are strikingly different as well. The patient is again dehumanized, developing some degree of social isolation and powerlessness in the hospital setting. I believe that personalized care, responsive to individual patient needs, cannot be provided without the nurse having some involvement with the person she is caring for.

But before she can decide on her philosophy of involvement, she must be aware of the side effects of that involvement. Her feelings may become apparent to the patient, other staff, and herself. More importantly, she will be open and vulnerable to more pain if she allows herself to feel with the person's condition.

I have chosen to disregard the traditional "professional distance" as I have worked with fatally ill patients and their families (and as I have worked with students, too). This has meant a great deal of effort directed toward developing the timing in the transition between involvement and objectivity. In addition, it has meant learning my own limitations and learning to be more careful about taking care of myself and meeting my needs in my personal life. Most of the patients I have become involved with have been children and adolescents, and I have experienced deep sorrow and grief many times. Fortunately, along with the pain, there have been many moments when I have felt very close to the most beautiful parts of whatever being human is about. For me, these moments and the insights I have gained into myself and life and death have made the painful feelings acceptable.

I have described how the overt expression of strong feelings is usually discouraged within our society. When we experience these feelings and deny them to ourselves, they interfere with our attempts to care for others. Once we face our own feelings of sorrow, anger, and guilt, can we share them with patients?

The major objection to professionals' expressing their feelings stems from the fear that they will fulfill their own needs rather than those of the patient. I agree that the aim of professional intervention must remain focused on the patient's needs; however, unless each nurse confronts and meets her own needs (this does not always take place within the context of the clinical interaction), she will be unable to continue to relate to others in any meaningful way. True, if the nurse breaks down crying uncontrollably, it may not allow the patient even to express his concerns or obtain help from her. If the nurse's needs in a work situation are too overwhelming to handle, she becomes responsible for obtaining help from other sources.

While I was looking over a chart in a ward setting, a new graduate nurse came up and asked for help. She had just gone through her first cardiac arrest, and it had been with a child she had cared for over an extended period of time. She told how she had managed to handle all the tasks that were required during the crisis; however, now the parents needed help and she felt she was too close to breaking down herself. She asked if I could stay with them. Later she expressed her guilt over "not being able to handle it." I saw her as handling it beautifully; when her feelings were so strong they threatened to prevent her from meeting the family's needs, she sought help from others. She sought support for her own needs afterwards and then was able to return to the situation.

This nurse recognized the limitations imposed on her by her feelings and was helped to see that it was both healthy and appropriate for her to grieve for a patient she had cared for. Enough support should have been given so that in future situations she will remain able to relate as a human, in touch with her experiences, feelings, and needs and always capable of preventing their interference with her professional functioning.

In other cases, when a patient talks of his impending death or the approaching death of a family member, the nurse may experience feelings of sadness that are not so overwhelming as those of the nurse just cited. What is the danger of sharing some of these feelings with patients and families? Again, this involves a decision each of us must make.

Very often in a situation where I have cared for a patient and family over a period of time, I have had tears in my eyes or cried quietly with the family after the death. What does this communicate? One mother expressed how important it was for her to see several of the nurses cry after her daughter's death. She felt it helped her realize that the people who cared for her daughter had cared about her as a person, and this seemed to alleviate some of the guilt she had been experiencing about the need to leave Lucy in the hospital.

I want to briefly explore another area connected with the feelings and involvement that arise from the problems of a helping relationship. Many nurses seem to need to "help" all the time. They feel good about themselves only as long as they can view themselves as helping others. While they view themselves as assisting another person, they feel they have control over the situation. If a person prides herself on control, expressing anger and sadness becomes especially hard.

Her feelings about herself come into focus here. Can she accept herself with all the feelings, both positive and negative, she has? If she does not see herself as worthwhile, can she risk talking to a patient without being certain she will hurt him? If she cannot accept herself, how can she really accept or like a patient? And, if she denies her own negative feelings, how can she be sensitive to those feelings in others? Unless each nurse works out some of these feelings about herself, and meets her personal needs outside the work situation, I do not believe she can work sensitively with patients, allowing them to live and die in their unique way.

REFERENCES

American Journal of Nursing Company Contemporary Nursing Series. 1972. *The Dying Patient: A Nursing Perspective.* New York: American Journal of Nursing Company.

Agee, J. 1963. *A Death in the Family.* New York: Avon. (Reprint of 1957 edition, New York: Obolensky).

Alsop, S. 1974. *Stay of Execution.* Philadelphia: J. B. Lippincott.

Benoliel, J. Q. 1970. "Talking to Patients about Death." *Nursing Forum* 9:263.

Choron, J. 1963. *Death and Western Thought.* New York: Collier Books.

de Beauvoir, S. 1966. *A Very Easy Death.* New York: C. P. Putnam.

Feifel, H., ed. 1959. *The Meaning of Death.* New York: McGraw-Hill.

Fletcher, J. 1973. "Ethics and Euthanasia." *American Journal of Nursing* 73 (April):670–75.

Fulton, R., ed. 1965. *Death and Identity.* New York: John Wiley.

Fulton, R., ed. 1973. *A Bibliography on Death, Grief and Bereavement: 1845–1973.* Minneapolis: University of Minnesota.

Glaser, B. G. and A. Strauss. 1965. *Awareness of Dying.* Chicago: Aldine.

Glaser, B. G. and A. Strauss. 1968. *Time for Dying.* Chicago: Aldine.

Grollman, E. A., ed. 1967. *Explaining Death to Children.* Boston: Beacon Press.

Gunther, J. 1949. *Death Be Not Proud.* New York: Harper and Row.

Jourard, S. M. 1971. *The Transparent Self,* p. 181. New York: D. Van Nostrand Company.

Kastenbaum, R. and R. Aisenberg. 1972. *The Psychology of Death.* New York: Springer.

Kubler-Ross, E. 1969. *On Death and Dying.* New York: Macmillan.

Lowenberg, J. S. 1970. "The Coping Behaviors of Fatally Ill Adolescents and Their Parents." *Nursing Forum* 9:279–87.

Neale, R. E. 1973. *The Art of Dying.* New York: Harper and Row.

Quint, J. 1967. *The Nurse and the Dying Patient.* New York: Macmillan.

Schoenberg, B. et al., eds. 1970. *Loss and Grief: Psychological Management in Medical Practice.* New York: Columbia University Press.

Solzhenitsyn, A. 1969. *The Cancer Ward.* New York: Bantam Books.

Strauss, A. L. and J. C. Quint. 1964. "The Non-accountability of Terminal Care." *Hospitals* 38 (January 16):73–87.

Sudnow, D. 1967. *Passing On.* Englewood Cliffs, New Jersey: Prentice-Hall, Inc.

Weber, L. 1973. "Ethics and Euthanasia, Another View." *American Journal of Nursing* 73 (July):1228–31.

Weisman, A. D. 1972. *On Dying and Denying.* New York: Behavioral Publications.

Wertenbaker, L. 1957. *Death of a Man.* New York: Random House.

11

Coping with Staff Grief

JAMES S. EATON, JR.

The care of the dying patient has become a subject of increasing concern to health professionals. Much of this interest has stemmed from the fact that more than 70 percent of deaths in the United States occur in hospitals—in settings where patients are removed from familiar surroundings of home, family, and friends—in settings where, not infrequently, physicians, nurses, and aides are the primary human contacts for the dying.

The recent recognition by nurses and physicians of their responsibilities toward the dying has prompted a growing body of literature in thanatology—the study of terminally ill patients and their families. It appears that insufficient attention has been paid to the peculiar stresses that affect the relationship between nurses and physicians when both attend a dying patient. Although each of our professions is accustomed to great responsibility for human life, only rarely do we recognize our mutual responsibility for providing an emotionally supportive environment in which not only the needs of dying patients are dealt with but also our own emotional needs are recognized and accepted when we are faced with the loss of a patient.

Nurses and physicians have long shared a difficult but honorable calling. To care for the ill and infirm, to treat and sometimes to save—these engagements have ennobled our professions and have enriched our lives. Somehow, the long hours, impossible schedules, and personal sacrifices along the way have come a bit easier with the knowledge that, by our hands and with our minds, human suffering is relieved.

But just as we share the common title of healer, so do we share common social and emotional vulnerabilities. Drug abuse and addiction, alcoholism, divorce, and suicide too frequently take their toll of our professions. Whether by occupational hazard or macabre twist of fate, these unfortunate vulnerabilities are perhaps more than coincidentally linked to our roles as healers—roles fraught with emotional demands.

Nowhere in our work are we more painfully aware of those demands than when we attend a dying patient and his family. It is in such a situation that a part of us seeks emotional support for ourselves from a fellow human being—as if to reaffirm our own quickness and life. But rarely do we communicate this need to each other.

Now, nurses and doctors do communicate. There is frequent colloquy between us in the nurses' station and around the ward desk; there is shared information on rounds; there are numerous orders and notes between us on charts, and more than a few telephone conversations. We are, indeed, colleagues and collaborators. Occasionally, we are lovers; frequently, we are friends.

How strange it is, then, with this common heritage and background and with this common dedication to our work, that, in the heavy presence of death, we are not emotionally drawn to one another more than either would have the other believe. This drawing together—if it occurs—would be an intensely human response, much the same as that of a person who, in the darkness of night, seeks out and is comforted by the mere presence of another human being. The loss of a loved one brings friends and family to the side of those who grieve. Indeed, the need for human contact and communication at such a time is universal. Why then are we, who after all are experts in the human condition, seemingly out of step with our fellow human beings when we must deal with death? Why do we so isolate ourselves from each other at precisely the time when isolation is counter to our deep emotional requirements?

The reasons, I believe, are complex. But they are worth exploring, for they may hold the key to improving the emotional health of our professions and, consequently, to improving service to our patients.

Somewhere in our training we have learned to hide feelings, to value detachment, and, above all, to present the posture of emotional aloofness in the face of death. But perhaps there are antecedent explanations also. Feifel (1963) postulates that one of the reasons people enter the healing professions is as an unconscious defense against inordinate anxiety about death—an anxiety that has its roots in childhood.

Other explanations must include the possibility that death for us is a defeat in our work to preserve life. Our narcissism and unconscious omnipotence are shattered when we lose a patient. Occasionally, also, the long terminal illness of a difficult patient has become so burdensome to us that, when the patient dies, nurse and physician alike feel a sudden relief—that sense of relief only to be followed by nagging guilt and shame, whenever its recognition erupts to consciousness. In short, there is probably no single best reason why death's sting seems to be more painful for doctors and nurses. That it is, however, seems to be manifested in our peculiar and sometimes poignant coping behaviors when dealing with the dying.

Black humor is just one of the ways in which our youngest colleagues defend against their strong anxiety in dealing with a ward of dying patients. More sophisticated, but still callous, behaviors of the more experienced in our midst include moving the terminal but still conscious patient to the end of a ward, behind screens; "forgetting" to make daily rounds on the dying patient; closeting ourselves away in nurses' stations or ward offices, feigning deafness to the occasional plaintive requests from dying patients; "allowing Mrs. Smith to rest, undisturbed" throughout a shift; and avoiding contact with the patient's family ("if patient expires, notify intern on call").

Unfortunately, both doctors and nurses occasionally indulge in laying unjustified blame for a patient's death at the feet of the other: "They shouldn't have tried that new medication on her . . . all it was doing was making her worse"; or "Why didn't you call me when he started going sour?"

This type of behavior is only another defense against our own uneasiness with death and is a projection to others of our own nagging questions of self-blame. Such feelings of self-accusation and recrimination are common when communication and open sharing of feelings are not possible between nurse and physician.

Another frequent and usually unconscious behavior that does us no credit is the tendency to approach the bed of a dying patient with our hands clasped behind our back, as if the time for "laying on of hands" or some other form of human contact had passed. The roots of these behaviors are to be found among the taboos of primitive peoples. And, like such taboos, our inappropriate mechanisms of defense against the fear of death fade when we begin dealing openly with the sources of our anxiety and when we can be part of a mutually enlightened and supportive professional milieu.

I do not wish to indict our two professions. Rather, I wish to call attention to the intensity of our anxiety over death and to the very humanness of our defense mechanisms. After all, we can never be blasé about death and still retain the humanist spark so vital to our continued function as healers of the body and mind. As long as human beings age and bodies go frail, there will be nurses and doctors. And as long as man is mortal, nurses and doctors will always need to cope with a patient's death and with their own anxiety over that death.

The relationship between ward nurse and doctor is strongly ambivalent. At times they are rivals for organizational power and for the respect of patients and other staff; at times they work in perfect social complement. A doctor gives orders to the nurse, and yet the nurse, more than any other person in the "system," runs the ward and provides the continuity of care, especially in a teaching hospital where house staff and faculty rotate ward assignments. The professional power or "clout" of the ward doctor pales against the stronger influence of the head nurse on the total operations of that ward. The nurse, then, is in the unique position for setting the "tone" of the ward and for taking needed initiatives in matters of emotional import among ward staff. A death on the ward is such a matter.

Frequently, staff have had to keep in check their feelings about a dying patient to help the patient and his family go through, at their own pace, the needed stages of recognition and acceptance. Then, after the patient's death and after dealing with the family, both nurse and doctor must come to grips with their own feelings about the loss of their patient. During this emotional catharsis, each must confront afresh his own mortality and the imperfection of medical knowledge. If one is to grow from such a cathartic experience, one must reaffirm his own personal and professional worth. Although these are largely unconscious processes, this is, nevertheless, difficult emotional work. We shirk from it and, if possible, leave the ward as quickly as we can, perhaps even denying to ourselves and to our colleagues that we have been very much affected by the death. But this emotional deceit does not fool us or our colleagues. Our grief work must be done if we are to maintain our emotional health and our professional humanism.

This professional grief work need not be of the same character, of the same depth, or of the same duration as that by the family or a loved one. More frequently, for us it consists of reminiscences about the patient, shared between nurse colleagues or between nurse and physician—what seemed "special" or unique about the patient; how the patient first came to the floor; how he will be missed by the food-cart man, or the aide on the night shift, and so forth. Sometimes our grief work is only a few moments of silence shared in the presence of colleagues. Sharing, here, is the important factor. The

emotional buttressing provided by another human being at
the time of our emotional vulnerability is vital.

John Bowlby, in his second volume of *Attachment and Loss*
(1973, p. 358) makes the point that:

whenever an individual is confident that an attachment figure will
be available to him when he desires it, that person will be much
less prone to intense or chronic fear than will an individual who for
any reason has no such confidence.

The point is made with particular reference to children but
seems equally applicable to the emotional needs of nurses and
doctors when they are faced with the unconscious "intense or
chronic fear" of death.

Early in my training, I cared for an elderly dying man
who, in his younger days, was a vaudeville performer and,
until his illness, a streetcorner tap dancer in the French
Quarter of New Orleans. He was one of those kind souls
who, although desperately ill, by force of his colorful personality, became a particular favorite of the ward staff. It was,
then, difficult for all of us to see this appealing little man
die—especially since his death followed close on the heels of a
series of probably unnecessary and painful procedures—cut-
downs, thoracenteses, tracheostomy, and so on.

During all of this, his meager family and colleagues were
in the floor lounge while a bevy of nurses and physicians
hovered about the patient's bed, imposing these somewhat
futile procedures on him. At the end, when, plain to all, he
was not to be resuscitated, we began to drift away. One of his
sons had been watching from the doorway—"Don't you all
leave yet," he said. And he came to the foot of his father's
bed along with the old man's dancing partner, his protégé.
Then, in the middle of this 12-bed open ward, with nurses
and doctors standing around a bit embarrassed and impa-
tient, the two mourners began a slow tap dance with tears
streaming down their faces, in tribute to the old man. Only a
few dry eyes were left when they finished a few minutes later.
But, with the necessary catharsis and brief grief work ac-

complished, the ward staff returned to their responsibilities with renewed purpose, with a reawakened sense of humaneness and, almost inexplicably, a bit refreshed.

Some may feel that this article has been a maudlin plea for the unleashing of rampant emotionality among professional staff at the time of a patient's death. This is not my message. Rather, I make a simple plea to our professions for a humanistic and thoughtful approach to the emotional needs of ourselves and our colleagues at a time of stress, especially at those times when death's sting pains us. Let us stop practicing emotional deceit.

REFERENCES

Bowlby, J. 1973. "Separation." In *Attachment and Loss,* Vol. 2, p. 358. New York: Basic Books.

Feifel, H. 1963. "Death." In *Taboo Topics,* ed. N. C. Farberow. New York: Atherton Press.

12

Pediatric Nurses Dream of Death

JOHN E. SCHOWALTER

DIFFICULTIES IN CARING FOR DYING PATIENTS

I have noted elsewhere that pediatric nurses must often struggle even more than doctors with their behavior toward dying
patients (Schowalter, 1971a). One reason is that they must
spend a relatively large amount of time with a patient while
having little or no say in decisions on the treatment regimen.
In other words, the nurse must carry out, and attempt to answer questions about, policy over which she has relatively
little power. Although this situation is often just as common
for less seriously ill pediatric patients, there is not around
these children the same aura of tenseness present in the rooms
of the dying. In addition, in the case of dying patients, questions are usually more hostile, physicians are often less available for backup, and answers are often less clear or pleasant.
It is well known that the fatally ill tend to be avoided, but
basic nursing care is "ordered," and at times, by ordering it,
physicians substitute nursing contact for their own presence.

A second difficulty for nurses working with the dying is
that their contact is so personal. It has to do directly with the

Supported by the Maternal and Child Health Division of the Health
Services and Mental Health Administration of the U.S. Department of
Health, Education, and Welfare; The Connecticut Department of Health;
and U.S. Public Health Service Grant No. 5T1 MH–5442–20.

patient's dying body and with his reactions to his medications and procedures. A mutuality, occasionally of hostility but usually of caring, develops that envelops the nurse in the fate of the patient. This is especially true in hospitals where an effort is made to provide continuity of care by reducing to a minimum the number of nurses who minister to a terminally ill child. This mutuality is usually a blessing for the patient but may be an anguish for the nurse. Two somewhat different factors seem to reinforce this bond. They are the length of stay in hospital before death and the number of discipline problems the patient presents.

The longer a nurse has known a child before his death, the more depressed she tends to be after that death. An apparent paradox we have found is that, the closer the contact a nurse has with a child, the less eager she is to agree with protracted attempts to prolong the patient's life once it is clear they will not be curative. This feeling often puts a nurse in conflict in university hospitals, where experimental treatments are not unusual and are important for research and where nurses usually have even less influence over policy than in private hospitals.

In 1917 Freud noted in *Mourning and Melancholia* (reprinted 1957) that ambivalence was of great importance in determining the difficulty a person has in mourning. When someone close dies, he wrote, mourning is more apt to be problematic if the survivor has mixed feelings about the deceased than if the feelings are quite purely positive or negative. This discovery of Freud's has maintained general acceptance, but only recently have I become aware of its relevance to certain dying patients on a pediatric ward—those who are complaining, demanding, or abusive and who set nurses to arguing among themselves in attempts to avoid being assigned to them. Although it is not uncommon for medical staff to be angry with the dying for not responding completely to their treatments, this emotion is usually not fully conscious. With the dying child who is difficult, a conscious feeling of dislike is added. There can seldom be pure dislike, however, since the nurse is under social and professional pressures to care, in both senses of the word, for her patients. As with children who are especially well known, the troublesome patient who dies often causes an inordinate amount of grief among the staff. Although relief is a common response in both instances, in the latter case there is usually considerably more guilt.

HOW NURSES CAN HELP THEMSELVES TO COPE

The obvious way to help nurses cope better with dying children is to have the physicians offer them not only support and understanding but also, as much as possible, a voice in the policy of the individual patient's care. We have facilitated this during the eight years' existence of the Adolescent Ward at Yale–New Haven Hospital through weekly staff meetings that focus on the psychosomatic issues presented by patients on the floor (Schowalter, 1971b). In these meetings nursing feedback to the housestaff and to the medical director of adolescent services allows joint decisions to be made on both the specifics and the philosophy of a patient's care. Because of my own interest and the sophistication of the staff, special attention is paid to the needs of the dying patient and of the individuals providing his care.

A second approach to helping nurses cope with the dying is having nurses help each other, and one aspect of this approach is the theme of this article. Each week, in addition to the psychosomatic staff meeting, I lead a meeting for the nurses as consulting child psychiatrist. The meeting is attended also by the ward social worker, recreational therapist, secretary, and teacher; the resident in child psychiatry assigned to the floor; and my research associate and any students in nursing, social work, or other disciplines working with patients at the time. It is, however, the nurses' meeting. The head nurse, in consultation with the others, sets the agenda. Usually, individual patients are discussed, but at other times specific topics are reviewed, role playing is done, or, perhaps most importantly, gripes, joys, and disappointments are aired. Since this meeting has been held regularly for eight years, it is conducted with a relative informality that is sometimes shocking to new participants. Nurses are encouraged to be frank with themselves and each other, and more than anything, the meeting acts as an officially sanctioned time for catharsis.

During one of these meetings, after a well-known and well-liked patient had died, a nurse remarked that she had dreamed about him the night before. To her surprise and that of the rest of us, a second nurse exclaimed that she had also had a dream about that same patient. As discussion about this phenomenon unfolded, it became clear that it was not uncommon for nurses to dream about patients before and after their death (Schowalter, 1973). In fact nurses' dreams were much more commonly about fatally ill children than about any others. My own curiosity was piqued, and I asked the nurses to write down and give me dreams they had about dying patients.

Since that time I have collected 20 dreams. A surprisingly consistent pattern is found in their manifest content. In all but two dreams either the dying patient was portrayed as well or a dead patient came alive. In one dream, occurring shortly after the nurse accompanied a dead 10-year-old boy to the hospital morgue, she dreamed of a dead old woman lying in a morgue who came alive and began to pursue the nurse. In another, a nurse dreamed that a dying child had already died. Although most of the dreams were frightening and the dreamer was awakened by her emotions, they were usually quite readily perceived as undisguised wish fulfillments fused with remorse and guilt about the lack of success the nurses had or were having with the child's treatment.

In many of the dreams the patient spoke. Intriguingly, the patient almost always asked something of the nurse. This was usually a question about the status of his illness or treatment, but at times was a request for a favor or a favorite food. The nurse often felt that being asked for something was a rebuke—as further evidence that she had not done enough for or given enough to the child.

Although I knew something about the personal lives of some of the nurses, no attempt was made to "analyze" the dreams in a pseudo-psychoanalytic way. Occasionally, a nurse would tell me individual associations, but for the most part the dreams, with the dreamers' permission, were used as vehicles for group associations during the weekly nurses' meetings.

Typical Dream Examples

A short while after Rocky, a 10-year-old boy, died of leukemia, a nurse had the following dream: "I was at my home. Rocky's mother phoned. She was very excited and said that Rocky was alive. When I said I couldn't believe that, she said she would have Rocky talk to me. He said it was true. A doctor in his country (he was not from the United States) had given him some new medicine to make him alive, and Rocky was going to come to the ward to prove it was true."

According to the dreamer, this dream was a turnabout in two ways. Rocky had come back to life, and the medicine that did it was from a doctor in his developing country rather than from the prestigious medical center he had traveled thousands of miles to be in. Doubts about whether or not care had been competently or completely given were often raised through the dreams. Another example of this is given below.

A nurse was caring for Stevie, a 13-year-old boy, on the day he died. What actually occurred was that, while he was in a high Fowler's position (sitting almost straight up), she put him under an oxygen tent and tucked the plastic around him. Although he was semiconscious and she did not want to leave him alone, she had to premedicate a patient who was about to leave for surgery. While doing this, she heard another nurse scream, "Stevie is on the floor!" By the time she got back to Steve's room, there was a crowd, and it was clear that he was dead. Although the resident assured her that Stevie must have died sitting up and then fallen, she felt terribly guilty. That night she had the following dream: "Stevie was in bed, and I kept trying to pull up the sidebar of his bed. The oxygen tent also kept falling off. The harder I would try to pull them up, the more resistance there was. I became frantic and repeated the action over and over until I awakened. That side of the bed was the same side as Stevie fell over."

Although it was usual for these nurses' dreams to bring a dead child back to life, a few of them also touched on what is a fairly common human fear, premature burial.

Kathy was a 14-year-old girl who, after a long illness, died of lymphoblastic leukemia. She was often in much pain and frequently cried out "Help me. Oh, help me!" While performing postmortem care, the nurse whose dream will be presented remembered remarking on how warm Kathy's body felt. Shortly after the death she had this dream: "Kathy died much as it had really happened. After I had put her in the shroud, I heard breathing sounds from inside. I called the resident, but he dismissed my story as 'impossible.' However, I went back and could now feel an apical pulse as well as hear breathing. I took off the shroud, and Kathy began to talk. I was so very happy she had life."

In the following three dreams, the dead child came alive, but before the dream's end, death and reality had again been reaffirmed.

The following dream was reported after an 11-year-old girl died of leukemia: "Debbie was in the dayroom and called me to bring her a glass of milk. (She enjoyed milk very much and frequently asked for it.) I gave her the milk, and she drank it. Then she sat down in a chair and said, 'Thank you. Now I can die.' Then she went on to die."

The night of the day a 12-year-old girl died of cancer, the nurse who cared for her had this dream: "Bobbi's mother phoned to say the girl wanted me to come to her house and see her doll collection. I did. Bobbi's room was in the attic, and all along the walls were shelves of dolls from all over the world. After a few seconds, Bobbi got out of breath and said, 'Oh, I have to lie down for a moment.' After she caught her breath, she asked me to stay a couple of days at her house. I looked at her and said, 'But Bobbi, you're dead!' At that Bobbi began to cry."

After the death of an 11-year-old girl, a nurse reported this dream: "I walked into Madge's room, found her dead, and went out to console her parents. Her parents claimed she wasn't dead and urged me to return to her room. I did, and she was sitting up, smiling and talking. I returned to the parents, and then they entered Madge's room. They came out crying. She was dead. At this point I woke up."

The final example is about a troublesome patient of the type mentioned earlier. Arnold had a very serious heart block and ventrical septal defect. His cardiac pacemaker was malfunctioning, and he was considered close to death. He was also extremely difficult to nurse. He complained constantly and knew he was disliked by nurses and fellow patients alike. In the dream he died, but the nurse, stung with rebuke, resurrected him and reasserted her dedication.

During this hospitalization, there was much questioning about whether or not a new cardiac pacemaker should be implanted surgically into Arnold's heart wall and what his chances were to survive such surgery. After a number of changes of mind, the surgeons decided that the procedure would be too risky. The nursing staff had hoped the surgery would be tried, since they believed it was Arnold's only hope for survival. It was at this time that a nurse who often cared for Arnold had the following dream: "Arnold arrested. All the nurses, doctors and other staff were in his room trying to revive him. One of the doctors pronounced him dead. We all walked out not saying a word. Some of the other nurses and I went back to get his belongings together. When we walked into the room, he sat up and said, 'Please don't give up on me. Even though you don't like me, please don't give up. I'm still alive.' I awoke screaming, 'Don't give up!' "

Associations

Although nurses would occasionally speak to me privately about their dreams and ask my opinion of them, dreams were usually discussed by the group. When nurses had dreams about dying or dead patients, they wrote and gave them to me. There was, of course, an obvious selection process, since some relevant dreams were undoubtedly forgotten, others were not recognized because of their complexity, and still others, perhaps, were consciously withheld. When a nurse did report a dream, she was asked if she would mind if I read it for group associations. On two occasions I was asked not to present the dream. Permission was obtained from both the dreamer and the persons associating to present this material for publication.

Below are a few excerpts of comments as examples to show how the group process works.

To the dream mentioned earlier about Rocky, who came alive in his native country, the nurse who helped the dreamer prepare Rocky after death recalled that at that time the nurses questioned whether he was really dead. She recalled it this way:

We washed him up and wrapped him in the shroud. He was on an air mattress at the time, and when we turned him, there was a sound just like he breathed. The two of us just looked at each other wide eyed and we had to unwrap the shroud and prove to ourselves that he really wasn't alive.

There was then a general discussion about the common fear that patients will be taken to the morgue while still alive. A number of nurses said they often listen again for heartbeats even on the way to the morgue. Another nurse recalled her feelings toward Rocky's parents when they insisted that every medical measure continue, and his death was, as a consequence, prolonged and very painful.

Rocky was really and truly suffering, and yet the doctors were doing this and doing that. He was getting all kinds of medication, and I really got mad. I wanted him to live, but not that way. That wasn't living; it was pure hell. Yet at the same time I have another difficulty. I walk into a room and wonder if the child is alive. I find out he is comatose, but then in a very short time when I come back or even while I'm there, he is no longer alive. That's a body there but not a living thing anymore. Each time I have to pound it into me what happened, but how can such a big thing finally happen in just a brief second?

Another nurse added:

I'm Catholic and kind of religious, but I get angry that when someone is dying he loses his own personal sense of dignity. It seems they do all these torturing things to you that they would never dare to do to someone healthy, and it isn't just to save a life because a lot of times we know it won't. I don't know how to explain it, but with chest tubes coming out of you and all kinds of holes in you, you just become a mangled thing of sorts. I can just hope that they are suffering hell now and that death is kind of a release from this hell. That's the only way I can reconcile myself to the death of a child and that isn't too easy either.

Much feeling then was expressed about the seeming injustice of death during childhood and before fulfillment.

In the meeting in which the dream about Arnold was discussed, the problems involved in caring for a child who was both dying and unlikable were aired. It was noted that, although nurses often hoped for a child's death and almost always felt guilty for this wish, there was a much worse feeling present when they knew they did not like the patient and might be wishing in their own interests rather than in the interests of the child to end his misery. In short, it was the difference between associating oneself with murder as against euthanasia. As one nurse put it:

When you don't like a kid who's dying and you know you're working with him, it's really hard to get up and get in to work in the morning. It's like it's more than just two separate things, but as if they climb on each other to make one gigantic problem. The scariest part is what if you want them to die? Or, does even wondering if you wish it mean that you really do? You know in your mind that your wishes don't have any power anyway, but in your heart you're not so sure, and it makes you feel like a rotten person.

Other nurses said that they had the same worries, especially when they were alone off duty and were thinking over what happened during the day. Another wondered if they would worry so much about these patients if it was not for the nurses' meetings. Almost everyone agreed, but the consensus was that the feelings would probably be there anyway and that it was better to know what was bothering them than remain unfeeling and ignorant.

A final example of group discussion followed the dream mentioned earlier, the one that involved not a child but the old woman in the morgue. The dreamer described having

heard a scream and turned to see the dead woman pull off the sheet and start to get off the table. I let out a terrifying cry since the woman had a determined look on her face and I feared she was going to get me. Some pathologists heard my cry and rushed into the room. I remember feeling that because of their reaction what was happening must be true. I woke with the sensation of running, screaming, and trying to get away

The dreamer's associations had to do with the death during her childhood of a beloved great-aunt, but the dream touched on a number of professional concerns for the other nurses. Thoughts began with the morgue.

You just go into this room and there are shelves. A fellow human being whom you cared about and you just kind of cart them down there and shove them in a freezer. You just close the door and that's it. It's just such an empty feeling.

Another nurse added:

What really hit me the first time I took anyone to the morgue was that the stretcher they use doesn't have any padding on it. You suddenly realize you're no longer treating that person as a human being. What I heard in the dream was sort of an angry response in a corpse coming to life and chasing you because of what you're doing to them or have done.

"Every time I prepare a patient with a shroud," continued a third nurse, "I always feel that this is going to happen to me some day and will I want someone to put a shroud over my face? Automatically, I treat the body with more respect." Yet another nurse spoke of feelings of anger and resentment:

Just after a death I have to really watch myself, my attitude toward other people. It usually doesn't go on for a long time, but without guarding myself I become very angry with everything around. In nursing school they teach you that you are the professional who can't show emotion and whom others lean on. They also teach you that sadness and grief are the standard reactions of society to death. Well, all this flying back and forth makes you mad because you must act one way when you feel the other way. I know that I spend more time with healthier patients after someone dies. I don't want to get close to someone who is really sick. I want to see healthy people. I want to see people with life in them.

"It's not all bad though," the third concluded:

I think you learn to really appreciate life more from being a nurse, from watching people die and from thinking about it. You may not be happier than other girls, but you appreciate just the fact that you can get up and be healthy in the morning. After a death I'm much more appreciative of the relationships I have and the people I'm with—that they're alive and I'm alive. I think the nursing we do gives us an added dimension, for better and for worse, that other people can never know, and it makes you much more keen on what life really is.

CONCLUSIONS

Nurses are thrust into a very difficult position by having to provide intimate care for dying children while usually having relatively little influence over the treatment philosophy or regimen. A number of approaches have been used to aid nurses in becoming more active participants both in decisions about patient care and in helping each other cope with problems specific to the dying. To the second point and within a setting that involves a continuing group process, nurses' dreams have provided a unique tool for use in understanding the impact and the difficulties of working with dying children on an adolescent ward. Although representing only one of many ways to explore nurses' feelings about their work with dying patients, at least five advantages have accrued from this particular experiment.

1. The use of dreams to explore feelings about death provides the researcher with yet another window through which to view caregivers' reactions to the dying.

2. Dreams provide the nurses with materials, often otherwise unconscious, that express their feelings about stresses current in their work with dying patients. Bringing these feelings into consciousness makes them accessible to be dealt with by the individual and by the group.

3. The use of group associations allows others in addition to the dreamer to understand and expand their thinking about the practical and philosophic aspects of caring for the dying. The group experience provides not only the cognitive input of others but also the realization that others wrestle with and are frustrated by the same universal and not easily solvable psychologic tasks. This realization and feeling of community can be very comforting.

4. This approach has allowed us to learn something about dreams. Following the external stress of caring for a dying child, the manifest content of these dreams is quite simple. Almost without exception it includes the wish fulfillment that the child recover and is mixed with guilt that the nurse had not done as much for the patient as she should have. The dreams are similar to those following traumatic events, as reported by others.

5. Finally, the personal quality inherent in dreams seems to enhance the effect of their discussion on the discussants' personal lives. It was clear for many nurses that, as through any serious approach to understanding death, the examiners end up with a better understanding of life.

REFERENCES

Freud, S. 1957. "Mourning and Melancholia," pp. 243–58. In *Standard Edition*, Vol. 14. London: Hogarth Press.

Schowalter, J. E. 1971a. "Death and the Pediatric Nurse." *Journal of Thanatology* 1:81–90.

Schowalter, J. E. 1971b. "The Utilization of Child Psychiatry on a Pediatric Adolescent Ward." *Journal of the American Academy of Child Psychiatry* 10:684–99.

Schowalter, J. E. 1973. "The Experience of Death on an Adolescent Pediatric Ward." In *The Child in His Family*, ed. E. J. Anthony and C. Koupernik, pp. 211–18. New York: John Wiley & Sons.

13

A Personal Perspective of Death and Dying

LIBERTY KOVACS

IN MEMORIAM

Joe had been a patient for 25 years when I met him. As a young man he had come to this country from Poland to work in the coal mines of a midwestern state. Here is how he described it:

My life was very short. I was 17, and all my life I had been half-starved. Now, I had work in the mines—all the work I could do—12 hours a day. Six months later, there was an explosion in the mine. My friend was killed, and my back broken. I've been here ever since. The miner's welfare is paying my room and board. I had no place to go, and the hospital is as as good a place as any. Besides, my life stopped there in the mine, so what difference does it make?

The incoming students had been cautioned by older students and nurses to "leave Joe alone. He's stubborn and aggravating. He insists on doing everything his own way—even his treatments." Even so, I made every effort to find time to talk with Joe. I didn't know why or what I wanted to accomplish, but we talked quite often during my next three years as a student nurse. I grew to like and respect Joe very much.

As time went by, his condition grew worse. Threats of

suicide were ignored. Joe wanted to die, and I felt distressed
and helpless. No one was doing anything. It was "just another spell" that Joe was going through. "Give him time;
he'll come out of it. He usually does."

One night on my rounds, I went to Joe's bed and touched
him lightly. "Joe," I whispered. He was too still. Suddenly,
I felt frightened. I pulled back the covers quickly and reached
for his wrist.

"Oh, Joe, what have you done!"

For an instant I stood there staring at the cut wrists, the
razor blades beside him, and the huge, liver-shaped clots.
There was still a pulse, but it was very weak. I ran to the
telephone and called his doctor. A sleepy voice answered and
in a quavering voice, I explained what happened. He
yawned—I could hear it—and precious moments passed before he said, "Get a type and cross-match for blood, call
surgery and tell them to get ready, and—oh, yes, give $\frac{1}{6}$
grain of morphine if he seems to be in pain."

I was shocked and hurt. No one seemed particularly disturbed. During report that morning, I stood sobbing uncontrollably.

"You should have given him more blades; he would have
done a better job then," remarked the nurse who relieved me.

Two days later Joe was transferred to the state hospital for
the mentally ill. He died there several years later.

In the years that followed, I learned to do what many people in the helping profession learn to do: switch off feelings
and dichotomize their lives—personal feelings get switched
off at work and professional experiences get switched off on
the way home. Needless to say, this solution takes a heavy
toll, recognized or not. Resolution of my experience with Joe
did not occur until 10 years later—during my own psychotherapy. I believe this dichotomizing process contributes to
the chronic dissatisfaction and demoralization so prevalent in
nursing.

Ignoring, avoiding, or trying to escape realities of life or death is not effective, as I came to realize eventually. The question becomes, "How can a nurse prepare herself to confront the realities of death (and of pain and suffering)?" Nursing education, in scattered instances, has begun to teach the psychological, social, and cultural aspects of death. Nursing service, with few exceptions, continues to regard death mainly as a physiological and technological process.

The alienation and dehumanization of the dying patient have been well documented. In the last decade a growing body of theoretical and experimental knowledge about death and dying has developed, all of it testifying to the fact that death can and must be approached more rationally and with better understanding than was available to me as a student and young graduate nurse.

PREPARATION

This article is my attempt to answer the question asked above: How can I prepare myself to confront the realities of death? The following discussion describes briefly the exploration of some of my ideas and experiences, and the influential social and cultural events that have provided me with a foundation from which I could *begin* developing a perspective of death and finding a place for it in my life as a person and a nurse.

Let me say here at the very beginning that I do not believe I have resolved all my fears and apprehensions about my personal death or about working with dying patients. These are but a few steps taken as preparation for moving more directly into the realm of death and dying with patients suffering from the more catastrophic conditions that befall human beings.

Although this exploratory approach is only one way, I am convinced that multiple pathways to learning about and confronting death are available to those willing to search for them. When I started this journey, I discovered that throughout my life many opportunities to *think* about and *respond* to death presented themselves to me—if only I could allow myself to acknowledge my experience with death.

Kubler-Ross (1969) suggests that "we should make it a habit to think about death and dying occasionally . . . before we encounter it in our own life" (p.26). In ancient Rome, charioteers were reminded by slaves, *"memento mori"* (remember you must die). Since I drive the freeways daily, I remind myself of this. Needless to say, much conscious effort is required to overcome the resistance to even thinking about death, for as Freud (1920) pointed out, "unconsciously . . . everyone of us is convinced of his immortality" (p. 50).

Talking with dying patients is the most direct way to learn what death means and how patients respond to dying. This approach requires that the nurse be prepared to deal with the emotional impact of this encounter with at least one other person who is willing to listen and explore thoroughly the interaction that took place with the dying patient. This process within a process (nurse–patient and nurse–consultant) has benefits of fulfillment and meaning, not only for the nurse but also for the patients and their families. Rather than concerns about "not enough time" or energy, the nurse gains a sense of achievement, and the patient a sense of dignity as a human being. Both win.

Exploring literature may be less direct, but I think knowing others' experiences, theories, and views is a necessary adjunct to one's own experience and knowledge and helpful in developing a philosophy of life that includes death.

The other directions may include talking with members of dying patients' families, or with staff, students, and coworkers who are working with dying patients or who may themselves have a family member who is critically ill.

As a teacher and consultant, I have learned, and am helping students and nurses to learn, about a wide range of emotional states: anger, hostility, aggression, and joy, as well as the more poignant feelings of loss through separation and death that we may encounter in our professional and personal lives.

Still another pathway that may be taken is introspection—
the examination and review of the experiential, social, and
cultural influences in one's personal life. I believe this direction is important if a thorough integration of theoretical
principles and concepts is to take place. Without this experiential factor, intellectualization may be the final result.

I remember during my early years that death seemed an
unavoidable and inevitable force. As children, my brothers,
sisters, and I were involved in all events, whether these were
weddings, baptisms, or funerals. Although funerals were
heavy emotional experiences for adults, children were not
shielded from them. Death was approached in a ritualistic
way that provided built-in supports and structure for all who
participated in the funeral and the mourning process afterward. In this way, the deep sense of loss could be experienced and shared completely.

In everyone's life there are social and environmental realities that are difficult to escape. In my own life, growing up
near the banks of the Ohio River, drownings of friends and
acquaintances became a dreaded event almost every summer.
With steel mills, blast furnaces, and coal mines nearby,
death hovered over our valley constantly, for mines and furnaces have a tendency to explode, and men were injured and
killed.

Although death was a fearful and tragic event and often
appeared out of nowhere like a malevolent monster, it was
also viewed as an awesome reality that everyone was expected
to confront sooner or later. Being aware of the existence of
death and participating in the rituals and the mourning gave
order and meaning to loss through death.

Not until my entrance into a school of nursing were conflicts aroused in me about the emotional aspects of patient
care. Before this time, I viewed emotions as natural responses
to life situations; in nursing, however, they were considered
irrelevant and unacceptable. Rules and regulations established the principle that emotional issues were not to be
discussed with patients (or faculty). Thus, faced with the rig-

orous demands and the anxieties of learning in the hospital and the classroom, suppression and control seemed the necessary means at that time. In many nursing situations, suppression and control are viewed as essential methods of dealing with painful issues such as death. However, when this is the *only* means available to nurses, dichotomization and isolation result, with negative effects for the nurse as well as for patients and their families.

Of course, each nurse must determine the impact of this approach for herself. Each nurse must make the decision about which direction she will take and evaluate the risks and outcome in terms of her own philosophy or frame of reference.

In my own experience, when I attempted to unlearn these latter influences and to get in touch again with the emotional aspects of my life, fears and apprehensions about "upsetting patients" and "making patients cry" had to be overcome. This unlearning process required certain intangible elements, such as acceptance, sharing, and acknowledgment, inherent in a functional teacher–student relationship, as well as theories, concepts, and principles from the behavioral sciences.

Again, I want to emphasize that the integration of the theoretical with experiential, cultural, and social factors can provide the nurse with a sound foundation from which to practice nursing most effectively, for credence and validity are given, not only to knowledge and technical skills, but also to life's experiences.

CONCLUSION

Let me conclude by sharing a couple of philosophical ideas, incomplete though they may be, that are strongly influential and basic in my work with people: My responsibility is to be available and to provide the conditions that will enable the other person (patient, student, nurse) to solve his problems and make his own decisions. He is responsible for choices that he makes in his life. I, as a professional nurse, am responsible for my part of the relationship: to listen, to try to understand, and to respond in kind.

This concept of responsibility (or "response-ability") has ramifications from birth to death. In relation to this discussion, however, I believe that a person has a right to decide how he will die. We must remember that people will die as they have lived. If they have denied problems, rejected responsibility for their thoughts, feelings, and actions throughout their lives, they will very likely do so on their deathbeds—unless they are assisted in learning new ways.

The value of this concept of responsibility for me has been a renewed sense of freedom in working with people. Now I can be with people with varying degrees of needs and problems and not feel obliged to carry the burden of solving all their problems or making decisions for them. I am available, attentive, and responsive—to what extent is strongly dependent on the patient's needs, willingness, and motivation to share in this proffered relationship.

Another idea I am trying to integrate into my practice is based on two compelling conclusions made by Freud and Jung. Freud (1920, p. 88) stated that "The goal of all life is death," and Jung (1959, p. 6), in a gentler way, commented, "Only he remains vitally alive who is ready to die with life." More recently, Kubler-Ross has suggested that professionals be available to help patients "die by trying to help them live" (1969, p. 21).

Although I am not convinced that the goal of my life is ultimately death, I can accept the fact that the striving, searching, and struggle—the pain and joys involved in these efforts—will culminate in my death. Hence, the realization arises that the unconscious desire to *overcome* and *prevent* pain, suffering, and death, implicit in the attitudes of many helping professionals, may be an unrealistic and impossible task that we set for ourselves. Beyond that, abolishing pain would be undesirable; pain is a necessary condition of growth, innovation, and creativity. The fallacy of our age is that life without pain is possible.

Rather than expending so much energy in avoidance, denial, and escape tactics, let us instead make room in our view of life for pain, suffering, and death. Accept the fact that these aspects do exist, and are relevant and accessible to confrontation and management. Knowing and accepting these facts of life can pave the way for working with greater equanimity in helping to relieve some of the pain and suffering and in being able to offer hope, meaning, and dignity to those facing death.

REFERENCES

Freud, S. 1920. *Beyond the Pleasure Principle.* Trans. James Stachey (1950). New York: Liveright.

Jung, C. G. 1959. "The Soul and Death." In *The Meaning of Death,* ed. H. Feifel, p. 6. New York: McGraw-Hill.

Kubler-Ross, E. 1969. *On Death and Dying.* New York: Macmillian.

14

Female Chauvinism in Nursing

JOSEPH F. FENNELLY

The nurse must change her role in and her position on the medical team that gives care to the dying and suffering patient. Many of the patients' needs are denied them because the nurse rejects her role as a prime mover on the medical team and, even if reluctantly, relinquishes her responsibility to someone else, usually the physician. Further, because the nurse pictures herself as a member of a team in which there is a hierarchy, much of what the patient says is filtered out, and no meaningful medical intervention or environmental change is therefore effected. The nurse must reexamine her role in the light of meaningful change.

There are forces that are keeping the health team members apart. Each element of the medical system is constantly undergoing change. Change is encircling and engulfing us like atoms knocking and hitting into other atoms but not merging together.

There is little need to dwell on the changes within nursing. We could point to them in many areas—the academic, the various professional organizations, the number of years required to receive the R.N., the nursing specialist, the licensed practical nurse, and so forth. To confuse matters more, we now have the "physician's assistant." In an article in *Nursing Digest* (February 1974), Trucia D. Kushner attacks the concept of the physician's assistant as an attempt to reduce the nurse to a lesser role. It is not unfair to say that Ms. Kushner's viewpoint is derived from the feminist movement.

The changing concepts of physicians' training can fill volumes, and there is no need to quote references here to appreciate the variations and changes in the structure of the doctor's educational program.

The role of the "paraprofessional" (a term that I do not appreciate in concept but only as a specification of a group important to the patient) also needs definition. The paramedic, the occupational therapist, the inhalation therapist, the physical therapist—all are also involved in the care of the patient, and again, their roles are somewhat poorly defined.

Next, one has to include the hospital environment, the problems of hospital administration, and the constant struggle to designate who is in charge. The power struggles of the hospital staff, the hospital administrators, the doctors, and the nurses affect each person to a greater or lesser degree. Needless to say, the role of government and nongovernment in terms of controls and third-party payment increases the number of people involved in the care of the patient. (Little wonder that medical care today is the second biggest industry in the country.)

A case report demonstrates the problem. A patient in her late fifties was admitted to the hospital with what was originally diagnosed as a potentially curable cancer of the uterus. Approximately four months before her admission a surgically correctable condition, a lesion in the right kidney artery, was found that caused sustained and severe high blood pressure. For reasons not germane, the kidney lesion was not interrupted or cured surgically, and resulting cardiovascular disease with heart failure developed. When the patient was admitted to the hospital with the carcinoma, there was also an underlying severe metabolic disease that necessitated a strict low-salt diet to prevent fluid retention and additional heart failure complications. The carcinoma was felt to be inoperable by virtue of its spread beyond a resectable surgical lesion; a curative dose of cobalt X-ray therapy was therefore started.

During the therapy, there were frequent symptoms of bladder spasm, abdominal pain, and severe diarrhea. The patient's appetite was reduced markedly. She developed a fixation on grape juice, and the staff became locked in a battle to get more nutritious foods into her.

Approximately three months after the treatment had begun, an eminently warm nurse walked up to the doctor and said, "Doctor, the patient is angry with me because she is tired of our making her eat this bland, low-salt diet, and, further, I don't like the patients to be angry with me. It upsets me." With some hesitation and minor trepidation, she added, "Doctor, the patient keeps asking for a bacon, lettuce, and tomato sandwich. Would you mind if we gave her this sandwich?" With this, the doctor saw a striking picture. He asked himself *"My God! What is this patient being treated for?"* He realized that the hospital was treating something in the patient, but was not treating the whole patient. So he said, tongue in cheek, "What are you trying to do to my patient? You know she has high blood pressure, and bacon has too much salt, and salt is bad for high blood pressure." He added, "Nurse, don't you realize that I try to be a complete doctor and recognize the patient's needs and treat the whole patient and have a good bedside manner, and even try to hold her hand and speak to all her needs?" (He realized that despite all of his fantasies about what kind of doctor he thought he was, the conditioned ingrained concept "treat the lesion" had pervaded his thinking.)

He went on: "Nurse, what took you three months of struggling to suggest to me that she have a bacon, lettuce, and tomato sandwich? After all, she has an unresectable, incurable right renal artery lesion; she has little hope of a cure. Furthermore, she has been in this hospital for three months, no family has visited her on any regular basis, she has adopted this ward as her family and her home, and yet we miss the forest for the trees. And despite the fact that I have tried to communicate these facts to the staff, we deny her this pleasure." The patient was given her sandwich; afterward, her mental attitude improved, and her blood pressure was no more difficult to manage.

I am chagrined that, because of the restrictions of "proper care," this patient was denied many days of pleasure; she died approximately three months later, after going through many necessary therapeutic endeavors that provoked a good deal of pain and suffering.

What are the solutions in terms of the concept of female chauvinism? The traditional training of the physician is geared to technicological expertise, but during this long training period, the teacher, the professor, has atrophied in terms of transmitting his personal feelings and his ability to use his total being as a tool of teaching. Consequently, the physician in training perceives his own role as one of treating the lesions expertly, in a scientific and categorical fashion. Unfortunately, he has not been taught by example from his teachers how to use his own being, his own humanness, as a tool.

But let us not again attack science or systems unless we can find solutions. Toffler (1970) postulates that technology itself has no moral or ethical value, or no intrinsic value system of superiority, and that it must be controlled by people. He further states that an "ad hocracy," a bringing together of capable people with a common goal, people who are experts, people who are not enmeshed in a hierarchy of responsibility, is one solution to this problem.

An excellent example of a system able to release technology is that of the problem-oriented medical approach. Although the progress of care in terms of our known deficiencies is painfully slow, Lawrence Weed (1973), in this problem-oriented system, has pinpointed some of these deficiencies, especially those centering around responsibility. He clearly suggests that the responsibility to the patient rests with each individual caring for the particular patient and that it is his or her responsibility to carry through to see that the patient's needs are satisfied.

An excellent example is the problem of a patient on welfare who was admitted to the hospital in need of a routine hysterectomy but who had, as another problem, a husband who was unemployed and a family who had not received the welfare check. The patient expressed great concern over this. The nurse automatically sought social work assistance, and by the third or fourth hospital day, when the patient threatened to sign out of the hospital because of her children's needs, the social worker was able to reassure her that the necessary funds were available to maintain her children during her long hospitalization.

If we can polarize the doctor as the "man in charge" and the nurse as the entire supporting system, from a conceptual standpoint we can make some observations that in no way will advocate the replacement of the doctor. There is nothing more satisfying to me than dealing with an informed patient and an informed, involved staff. (From a devil's advocate position, it is worthy of note that, deep down, the doctor knows he is not in charge anyway and that many of his decisions are controlled by many other circumstances and individuals.)

How can the nurse communicate? Again, the necessity for her to feel her responsibility in and of itself will provoke action. How that action is communicated, of course, is unique. The nurse as a "female" knows how to communicate to the doctor as a "male"—let me emphasize that I wish to intellectualize this concept—and the nurse can conceptually even "seduce" the doctor into her framework of thinking from a theoretical standpoint, just as the need to communicate to a dying patient may be on a sexual basis, at least in terms of total human sexuality.

I do not wish to become embroiled in the role of women's liberation, since there is a real need for all of us to redefine our sex roles, and as has been suggested, the women's liberation movement may be the way to do so. It may appear, however, that a certain amount of male chauvinism should enter this thesis. I am bold enough to suggest to the female and to the nurse that she has my blessing to take over. I am bold enough to suggest that I relinquish my role to her. Again, this is not the context of my thinking but only that the person in charge must be that person who is best equipped to handle the problem. Furthermore, there is no end to the need to communicate, and there is no quantum or quantity of information that cannot be intertwined in the total network of patient care to upgrade our *common* role. Although the health-care profession rests very heavily on a desire to serve other people and, hence, one's feelings are constantly involved in this, we must somehow be able to accept suggestions from individuals who are critical of us or who express themselves in a fashion that, perhaps, could have benefited from greater control of thought and more planning. Still, we must be mature enough to recognize legitimate criticism of our operative functioning or our failure to function.

Ultimately, our role as physicians and as professionals should be to assist the individual to be self-sufficient, if and when that is possible, just as a loving parent idealizes his or her role in "letting go" of a child.

The nurse who eludes the patient's problem as "not my responsibility" is being as chauvinistic in her responsibility as the physician who rejects the patient's problem because he does not see it. Not only is the nurse denying the patient, she is constricting her own experience, her capacity to give herself to her profession and grow with it accordingly.

As long as each and every society, from the Stone Age society of the Tasadays to the nuclear society of today, remains wed to the necessity that no man is an island and each man's loss is felt by every man, then we can accelerate the "post-nuclear society" toward a fuller experience of the positive results of giving ourselves to others. For somewhere enmeshed in our memories as doctors and nurses is the motivating reason for our choice—namely, to relieve pain and suffering. This is the *substance* of our charge to our society. Let us not become lost in the *form* of how it is done.

REFERENCES

Toffler, A. 1970. *Future Shock.* New York: Random House.

Weed, L. 1973. "Medical Education and Patient Care." *Medical Record.* Cleveland: Case Western Reserve University Press (distributed by Year-book Medical Publishers, Chicago, Illinois).

15

The Nurse in Thanatology: What She Can Learn from the Women's Liberation Movement

M. L. S. VACHON, W. A. L. LYALL,
and
J. ROGERS

In almost any discussion of the role of the nurse in the care of the dying patient one hears comments such as: "If only the doctors would let us, we could do so much more." "What can we do if the doctor won't tell the patient he's dying?" "Why can't the doctors be different?"

In the care of the dying as in many other areas of nursing the nurse fairly consistently seems to feel that everything would be perfect if only the doctor were different. We attempt here to look at some of the reasons why the nurse takes this stance. Particular reference is made to the effect this has on the nurse's role in thanatology. We then describe our work with a group of nurses in a cancer hospital and the significant insights gained during this experience that have relevance for nurse–physician relationships and the care of those with life-threatening illness. The article is predicated on the premise that, if change is to occur between physicians and nurses in thanatology, then it must be initiated by the latter, for the nurses, not the physicians, are displeased and complain about the current situation.

To gain a perspective on the nurse–physician relationship one must look briefly at the early socialization of the female.

(We assume that most nurses are females and most physicians male.) Bardwick and Douvan (1972) state that girls characteristically achieve in grade school because of the rewards they get for good behavior, rather than for the achievement itself. In adolescence, however, the establishment of successful, interpersonal relationships becomes the self-defining, most rewarding task, and at this point such qualities as independence, aggression, and competitive achievement, which might threaten success in heterosexual relationships, are largely given up. Females then tend to maximize their interpersonal skills and withdraw from the development of independence and competition.

Having been thus socialized, women tend to enter occupations wherein their skills of nurturance, empathy, and competence are used and aggressiveness and competitiveness are largely dysfunctional. Nursing can be seen to be almost prototypical of such an occupation. Indeed, studies of nurses describe them as having greater needs for affiliation, nurturance, succor, social control, and security than females in fields other than nursing (Mauksch, 1965). Their self-concept is said to be dependable, methodical, and conscientious, with a tendency to be submissive and to sustain subordinate roles. In addition they consider that in their role as nurses they are expected to be cooperative, considerate, conventional, and adaptable (Davis, 1971). Finally, they are found to be significantly lower in leadership and originality factors than women going into other occupations (White, 1973).

If nurses, as women, have indeed been socialized to consider the maintenance of smooth interpersonal relationships as a major function, is it any wonder that problems develop when the nurse attempts to cope with the greatest challenge to interpersonal relationships—the threat of death? The care of the dying person is fraught with difficulty since:

1. It challenges the nurse's need to nurture and be competent by presenting her with what is often regarded as a "therapeutic failure." Here is a patient who, despite her best efforts, will not live. She can at best only help him to die.

2. Her empathic sensitivity makes her particularly aware that the dying patient may be suffering tremendous anxiety, fear, depression, and anger. Because of her need to nurture and decrease psychic stress she is eager to help him to resolve his feelings so that he may die peacefully.

3. She becomes aware that part of the patient's problem may lie in the difficulty he is having communicating with his physician.

4. Her tendency to want to maintain harmonious relationships and not seem to be competing with physicians leads her to want to avoid confronting the doctor with what might be interpreted as criticism and a challenge of his medical management and/or judgment.

5. Her "feminine lack of aggressiveness" and desire to avoid leadership paralyze her so that she is unable to assume any initiative to remedy the situation.

6. She is, nonetheless, left with the tremendous anxiety evoked by her perception of the dying patient's needs, and to continue to function, she must dissipate this anxiety.

When nurses are confronted with such problems with dying patients, they often go through a standard repertoire of behaviors, none of which are very effective but all of which manage to dissipate some anxiety without seriously disturbing the status quo. The most common behavior is to damn the doctor and wish that he would change. Closely aligned to this is criticizing the hospital for allowing such situations to develop. One often hears such comments as: "This ward is supposed to be for active treatment cases; why don't they put all the dying patients some place else instead of making us waste our time on them?" Since hospitals do not usually isolate terminal patients, another technique nurses use is to isolate the terminal patient themselves. We are all probably familiar with the studies showing how nurses avoid answering the lights of terminal patients and place them in private rooms at the end of the hall farthest from the nursing station (Glaser and Strauss, 1965).

Frequently, nurses complain that they have made many

suggestions for change but "nobody listens." When such comments are further explored, it seems that the nurses have not followed up their criticisms or requests by formulating plans for positive action. The expectation is that others, notably the doctors, should take on the responsibility of facilitating and effecting changes, after first rewarding nurses with praise for bringing suggestions to their attention.

Since none of these above-mentioned techniques work really well and much anxiety still remains, nurses frequently resort to criticizing one another. Cleland (1971) speaks of the self-hatred seen so often in nurses, stating that it comes from the fact that women are taught from an early age how to lose gracefully and to acquiesce and please the master, who in this case is obviously the doctor. As the nurse learns how to fail by not criticizing or challenging the doctor and thereby allowing patient care to deteriorate, she learns to hate herself, and this hatred is then generalized to most or all other members of her profession. As a result we see the anger, bitterness, and frustration that often arise among nurses, especially when the stress of caring for dying patients becomes particularly acute. We also see large numbers of nurses leaving their profession, their idealism shattered.

We have then the problem presented by the early socialization of the female, compounded by the personality of the women so often attracted to nursing. Add to this the many ways in which nurses are further socialized so as to enhance their basic tendency to avoid risks and self-exposure: to faithfully carry out prescribed tasks without the discretion normally accepted in most situations of responsibility (Menzies, 1961), and to believe that rebellion violates not only her professionalism but also her very feminity (Ehrenreich and English, undated). Is it any wonder then that we run into the problems we do with the dying patient?

Confronted with such a situation and aware of some of the stresses they were experiencing, one group of nurses decided to act. They worked in a cancer hospital, and so were constantly exposed to the stresses inherent in caring for patients with life-threatening illness and watching some of them die. The nurses had ineffectually tried to get help before, but nothing had ever happened. At one point, when confronted with a number of particularly stressful deaths, increasing staff conflicts, and the feeling that doctors were not being sufficiently supportive, they decided to demand help instead of resorting to their usual passive complaints.

A petition was drawn up asking for a psychologist or psychiatrist to help the nurses deal with dying patients. The petition, signed by all the nurses in the hospital, stated that, whereas they had previously dealt only with the physical needs of the patient, they were now attempting to meet the patient's psychosocial needs as well and were becoming increasingly aware of their inability to do so. They felt this inability stemmed from a natural fear of illness and death, a lack of knowledge and skill in interpersonal relationships, and a lack of communication skills. In addition intensive contact with patients and families made them acutely aware of the stresses both were experiencing, but because of a lack of resource personnel, they had to deal with these problems on their own, and this led to dissatisfaction in all concerned (*Petition,* 1971).

The petition was brought to the nursing and medical directors of the hospital, and the services of the two senior authors were obtained from a nearby psychiatric institute. Each of us met weekly with the nurses on two units for successive periods of eight weeks until all the nurses in the hospital had had the opportunity to attend the series of group meetings. Our general goals relative to the nurses were the following.

1.   To facilitate communication among the nurses, between nurses and patients, and between nurses and other professionals.
2.   To decrease the discomfort in discussing matters related to death and dying and increase the understanding of the feelings of staff and patients about this topic.

3. To promote increased emotional support within the nursing group and decrease reliance on doctors and others.

4. To promote an understanding and acceptance of the feelings of patients faced with life-threatening illness (Lyall, Vachon, and Nestor, 1973).

The groups focused on problems the nurses were having with their own feelings, with patient management, and with staff conflicts. Initially, we attempted to look specifically at the fears and problems presented by the dying patient, but it soon became obvious that this was not the most pressing issue. Rather, it seemed that the nurses were focusing on the problems in caring for the dying patient almost as a smoke-screen for more basic concerns. Gradually, working with the nurses, we were able to conceptualize their problems more clearly as follows:

1. The nurses had been well socialized to know that the "good nurse" never had "bad" feelings. As a result they were working in relative isolation, each one feeling she was the only "bad" nurse and the only one who at times felt angry, depressed, frustrated, helpless, and hopeless.

2. This led to mistrust among the nurses, who were hesitant to be open with one another for fear of criticism. As a result there was very little operative group support.

3. The lack of understanding and acceptance of their own feelings led to a lack of understanding and acceptance of the feelings of patients. In addition, the nurses were divided with respect to their feelings about the impact of cancer and the effectiveness of its treatment. The attitude ranged from: "Why do they bother taking treatment? They're only going to die anyway" to "Why should people be so upset just because they have cancer?" Conflict was compounded when patients were dying because the hospital was seen as an active treatment center and not a place where people came to die.

4. Because of the lack of insight into their situation, nurses were unable to function in their accepted role of maintaining smooth interpersonal relationships, and this led to anxiety,

which the omnipotent, omniscient physician was expected to resolve.

5. When the physicians failed to perform the expected magic and intervene to improve the situation, problems erupted, staff discord increased, and patient care deteriorated.

6. These problems all became particularly acute when patients in whom the staff had a significant personal investment were dying. In these situations the feelings of individual nurses were aroused, and they were unable to share them with one another; therefore they had trouble dealing with the patient and expected the doctor to help. He was often impotent, however, because of his own difficulties with dying patients. The nurses could not understand this because of the power and competence they projected onto the doctor.

It must be said that these problems were neither particular nor peculiar to the staff at this hospital. These nurses were, however, sufficiently responsible professionals to be willing to identify a need, ask for help, look openly at their problems, and attempt to find a solution.

It would be rewarding to report that the situation improved immediately after the groups were started. Such was not completely the case, but three years later, significant changes in the hospital milieu were still obvious.

As the nurses became aware of and began to accept their own feelings of anger, depression, frustration, hopelessness, and helplessness, they were able to share them with one another and receive support. This then freed them to use their natural empathy to accept and understand these same feelings in patients without feeling that they had to force patients to either repress or ignore their feelings for the expected smooth interpersonal relationships to occur.

Gradually, the nurses became at least able to entertain the idea that perhaps the physician might be experiencing some of the same feelings they had. At this point they were able to decrease their expectation of support from the doctors and began to feel that it might even be possible, through the support they gained from their own group, actually to be able to offer some help to the physicians in the grief they faced when patients died or were dying. This increased insight and also gave the nurses the initiative to approach physicians with the problems they observed and to suggest alternative approaches.

In view of the socialization process mentioned previously such independence, initiative, and aggressiveness are noteworthy changes for nurses. At times, however, their expanding role created difficulty because they had considerable ambivalence about accepting the responsibility that went with assuming initiative. It was much easier to criticize the doctor than to take the responsibility for initiating change. This was typified by one nurse who decided to question the physician's management of a particular patient. The doctor told her quite honestly that there was significant medical disagreement about whether this woman should have radical, mutilating surgery or should be allowed to die in peace. He was going to have to make the decision and was avoiding the woman because he didn't know what to say to her. At the end of the discussion the doctor seemed relieved to have shared his concern.

After the interview the nurse told the authors she had never realized "It was so lonely at the top." Always before she had naïvely assumed that doctors were omnipotent and knew what they were doing. She did not like knowing they sometimes had real doubts about the appropriate treatment for patients. This very competent nurse said she was considering resolving her conflict by never again questioning the doctor about his judgments.

Other nurses found pleasure in their new roles once they became aware that their skills were valuable and could be of considerable help to the physicians. For example, a nursing assistant and a resident went into the room to admit a 20-year-old boy dying of leukemia. The resident was unable to speak to the boy, whom all the staff had come to admire throughout his many hospitalizations. The nurse asked the patient how he was feeling and let him talk about his fears that this would be his last admission. She then stood aside expecting the doctor to take control. Gradually, she realized he didn't know what to say to the patient, and so she intervened and encouraged the young man to continue to express his fears, while she tried to offer him understanding and support. After they left the room, the doctor asked the nurse if she could help him to learn how to be as comfortable with dying patients as she obviously was.

Through our work with this group of nurses we all became increasingly aware of how the role and conflicts of the nurse mirror the role and conflicts of women in society. It also became obvious that these factors would have to be taken into consideration to effect change if the nurses were going to improve the care they were giving to patients.

By being willing to look at their own feelings and share them with their co-workers, the nurses gained new insights and strengths, similar perhaps to those gained in some consciousness-raising groups. This enabled them not only to increase their understanding of patients but also to expand their capacity to assume initiative and leadership in patient care. Relationships with physicians then improved because the nurses were able to realize that the doctors were also having difficulty in caring for dying patients. As pressures from the nurses on the physicians decreased, the doctors became much more willing to discuss treatment programs and to listen to the nurses' suggestions. This was not always easy for the nurses, because of the responsibility inherent in assuming initiative, and some nurses were sufficiently ambivalent about this new role for them retreat to their former passivity and the security of the status quo. For those willing to change, however, the rewards were great.

In conclusion, the authors would like to suggest that those in thanatology consider that the problems encountered in the care of the dying cannot be viewed in a vacuum but may, perhaps, be seen as being complicated by other issues of which we sometimes lose sight. In this particular instance the call for help in dealing with the dying patients masked a deeper problem of intrapersonal and interpersonal conflicts in the staff. Increased understanding of these issues significantly decreased the stress experienced in caring for the dying patients.

REFERENCES

Bardwick, J. M. and E. Douvan. 1972. "Ambivalence: The Socialization of Women. In *Readings on the Psychology of Women*, ed. J. M. Bardwick. New York: Harper and Row

Cleland, V. S. 1971. "Sex Discrimination: Nursing's Most Pervasive Problem." *American Journal of Nursing* 71, no. 8 (August):1542.

Davis, A. J. 1971. "Self-Concept, Occupational Role Expectations and Occupational Choice in Nursing and Social Work." In *The Professional Woman*, ed. A. Theodore. Cambridge: Schenkman Publishing Co., Inc.

Ehrenreich, D. and D. English. "Witches, Midwives and Nurses: A History of Women Healers." Oyster Bay, New York: Glass Mountain Pamphlets (undated).

Glaser, B. G., and A. L. Strauss. 1965. *Awareness of Dying*. Chicago: Aldine.

Lyall, W. A. L., M. L. S. Vachon, and C. P. Nestor. 1973. "Alleviating Stress in the Care of the Dying." Presented at Canadian Psychiatric Association's Annual Meeting, Vancouver, British Columbia (June).

Mauksch, H. O. 1965. "Becoming a Nurse: A Selective View." In *Social Interaction and Patient Care*, eds. J. K. Skipper and R. C. Leonard. Philadelphia: J. B. Lippincott.

Menzies, I. E. P. 1961. "Nurses Under Stress—3." *Nursing Times* (February 17): p. 206.

"Petition for Staff Psychologist," July 1971.

White, T. H. 1973. "Autonomy in Work: Are Women Any Different?" In *Women in Canada*, ed. M. Stephenson. Toronto: New Press.

16

Stereotyped Sex-Role Ranking of Caregivers and Quality Care for Dying Patients

NANCY PROCTOR GREENLEAF

The unexpected death of a patient admitted to the hospital for a routine procedure becomes part of the experience of those involved in the patient's care. It may trigger off acute grief reactions in all the staff. How well the caregivers can deal with these feelings has a direct bearing on the quality of care given the patient and family. If the staff retreat from themselves and each other, they can also be expected to retreat from the patient.

An example of this kind of situation is presented by a woman in her late forties who came to the hospital for a routine operation, common among people in her age group. The woman's heart stopped during surgery; no one was sure why. It became apparent that, before and during the cardiac arrest, the brain had had insufficient oxygen to sustain functioning. The patient was resuscitated and sent to the intensive care unit, where, after several days and three flat EEG's showing absence of vital brain function, all supportive therapy was discontinued with the consent of her husband.

Such a death is not routine. Yet many professional caregivers do have an experience with unexpected death in the course of their careers. Often such an experience leaves a deep and haunting impression on them, and rarely is there an opportunity to discuss and grasp the full significance of the event—one that produces a complex pattern of crises for the caregivers.

The focus of this article is on the interpersonal crises that an unexpected death precipitates for the caregivers themselves and on how it affects their shared experience, their humanity, and their ability to give intimate and compassionate care. Close examination of the caregivers' interpersonal relationships during and after an unusual experience with death is particularly helpful because the intensity of the situation exposes the flaws in their interpersonal gestalt. It is not business as usual but business at its most stressful. Each staff member become personally involved with the experience of loss, and each suffers his or her own special grief. The stress produced by this very human event exposes the constraints that sex-role stereotyping and ranking place on staff relationships and the resulting inhibition of compassionate caregiving. The doctor and nurse are typically locked into a hierarchical system wherein one always dominates the other. The patterns of interaction that develop in this ranking system are rigid and frustrate free exchange between people.

Several things happen in a crisis situation that affect the interpersonal gestalt of the caregivers. Two issues are particularly salient. One is the threat that emotionality and comforting seem to pose to the rational attitude that dominates medicine. There is a belief that strong, deeply felt emotions inhibit rational behavior and must therefore be repressed. The second issue considers the recognition of interpersonal needs in times of loss—needs that require an appropriate place within the work situation to be felt and shared. Such a place might be a health-team conference where interdependence of members is promoted and group leadership would vary, depending upon whose role most appropriately dominates in each situation.

The first issue deals with our human need for comfort.

When a small child stubs his toe and cries, mother comes and kisses it and makes it all better. What magic, and how we long for it at other times! We learn somewhere that mother's kiss can't always help, but the longing remains. We feel it in ourselves, and when we recognize it in others we feel sympathy. We wish we could reach out to others with a magic kiss or touch. Comfort is wanting to touch as well as wanting to be touched. It speaks to our longing for relatedness to others. We live in a culture that is uneasy with this notion, and the medical subculture seems to work hard to deny the very existence of such needs.

The second issue deals with interpersonal needs that can best be understood in terms of the dying child and her parents. The child desperately needs the parent to stay and give comfort. The parent, responding to the child, needs tremendous strength in the face of such a loss—a loss that must be experienced on some level as a terrible rejection. A part of all of us faces the death of a loved one with the same lonely confusion and sense of anger and guilt with which a small child experiences loss: I am accountable; I am bad; I did something wrong that is making this person leave me; I feel rage at being deserted. We understand the parent's need for large doses of caring and support from others. The parent leaves the bedside momentarily to be bolstered up and held together, and it is from the holding together by the intense caring from others that strength is gained—the strength needed to experience the event fully, to sound feelings, and to allow the comfort of others to touch us. Thus replenished, we turn to give our comfort to the dying—the person who is losing everything. We need others with whom to share our human feelings; that is how our humanity prevails, and yet it is in providing this caring, this holding together for each other, that the caregivers often fail. They fail because they are stuck into stereotyped roles ranked according to whose role is deemed most valuable, a phenomenon totally irrelevant in the tragic situation. The patient, family, and staff form a group of people who must say goodbye to one of the members of the group. Such a human event should not be burdened by role ranking.

One way of looking at the difficulties that role stereotyping and ranking produce is to consider the situation where death has become inevitable. In such a situation, curing is no longer possible and the need for caring becomes dominant. Caring is the province of nursing, and yet clearly it is the doctor who is in charge of our medical universe. The feminine, mothering nursing role is not allowed to emerge as dominant. The male, medical role dominates always; nurses work under "doctors' orders." What the nurse contributes independently seems little recognized or supported. I suspect that what happens when the nurse role becomes appropriately dominant is that the doctor feels useless because his leadership role is no longer necessary, and so he withdraws. The nurse, on the other hand, needs the continued support of the doctor and the rest of the staff to bolster her and help her find the strength to remain in intimate contact with the patient. She does *not* need to feel that her contribution is devalued or that she is abandoned by attitudes like those reflected in the following comment: "The only thing we can do for this patient is to provide good nursing care, so let's leave the nurse alone so she can give it." Rather, she needs to have recognition from the doctors that her role matters very much and that they, understanding the importance and difficulty of her task, are ready to stay with her, to stand behind her, and to support her. Leaving the nurse to face the experience alone simply results in her impoverishment; she then withdraws from the dying patient. It is the notion that the male-doctor role always and exclusively leads and that the female-nurse role always and exclusively supports that prevents the doctor and the nurse from attaining true colleagueship. The patient ultimately loses in a system where the interpersonal relationships of the staff become so unfulfilling. Unable to replenish themselves, the staff members withdraw from each other and the patient.

In my capacity as a psychiatric clinician in a general hospital, I set up weekly conferences with the staff nurses on the intensive care unit to discuss whatever issues are relevant to patient care. It took nearly 18 months to break through various barriers to these weekly conferences. The nursing leadership of the unit was very wary of the meetings and what they might accomplish. There was an attitude that dealing with feelings would be too stressful and that it was better to "let sleeping dogs lie." They needed time to develop trust in the clinician's motives. Nursing administration had to deal with the need for adequate staffing without which time could not be allowed for conferences. The unit instructor should be given credit for helping to break through the resistance by helping others recognize the need for conferences and by encouraging staff participation.

When the above-described unexpected death occurred, a natural forum then existed where nurses could share their deep grief. Their comments speak eloquently:

That poor doctor so needed to be helped; he was just beside himself with grief.

I felt like an accomplice, even though I knew it wasn't so.

I so wanted to be able to say something to the doctor to make him feel better.

I desperately needed to talk to someone. I kept choking up.

Every time one of her children would come in to see her they would look at her, all connected up to the machinery, totally unconscious, and they would become hysterical with grief—and so would I.

I was afraid I wouldn't be able to take care of the other patients.

When I finally got myself together enough to express my deep sympathy to one of the doctors, he said, "that's okay, you're only a nurse."

"That's okay, you're only a nurse!" What can that mean? It must mean something for, in fact, it is not an uncommon expression. When someone reaches out to us in our grief, we do not usually say, "That's okay, you're only a person." It is doubtful that a similar comment is ever made to a doctor. The message cannot escape us. *He responded to her status and thereby devalued her offering.*

The estrangement that occurs with role ranking is further exemplified in the following comments: "The doctor came to me after it was all over and said 'thank you.' I was surprised. I wanted to respond to him, but I felt so cut off from him that I just couldn't." She felt cut off because her sense of self-worth relative to his seemed so insignificant to her, and a part of her hates him for that—not purposefully and consciously but nonetheless pervasively.

"It was late in the evening, and some of the doctors were in the conference room talking about what had happened. I felt lonely and wanted to join them and share some of my own deep feelings. I kept walking by the door, trying to hear what they were saying. I felt silly for doing that, but it was my experience as well as theirs." Why could she not take some initiative and go into the conference room? Why was she not invited in? The answers to these questions seem to be that the type of sharing going on required a sense of colleagueship and could not reach through the barriers that ranking imposes.

The input to the staff in such a crisis must come from the professional group working together. The intensity of the circumstances simply does not permit casual discussion in friendship and family groups outside the medical community. Moreover, the sharing needs to occur with others intimately involved in the experience. Interdisciplinary conferences, established to deal with all aspects of patient care, would build a sense of trust and support and establish a forum where caregivers could pull together to meet their own interpersonal needs in a time of extreme stress.

The problems stemming from sex-role stereotyping and ranking are often and erroneously attributed only to the members of the dominant role. In fact, the change toward a more humane attitude about ourselves and the patients we care for must come from all concerned with good care. The discomfort with an appropriate dominance of the female-nurse role is felt by both doctors and nurses. It must also be realized that the image of total, godlike omnipotence is as much of a burden for doctors as the handmaiden image is for nurses. The problem belongs to all caregivers.

The approach to remedying the situation needs to be inter-disciplinary from the onset. Krant (1972, p. 101) notes that "an interdependent flow of information, decision sharing and care giving among staff members is essential to any attempt to alleviate the psychological and socio-economic problems that weigh on patients and families, and on staff as well." Krant continues:

Initially we attempted to loosen the dominance of the doctor in relation to others. This doctor dominance could not be done away with entirely, but a system of peer relations was innovated in which doctor, nurse and social worker were assigned equal status in data gathering and decision making as part of a creative learning enterprise. The physicians, especially the house officers, were asked to accommodate to the rearranged professional order. Nurses, so-cial workers, aides and others were encouraged to give their opin-ions and judgments openly and to feel qualified to offer ideas for designing as well as giving care and to raise issues (Krant, p. 102).

The contrivance of this structured "interdependence" simply emphasizes the pervasiveness of the problem. It says we can work together as autonomous contributors to a team when a member of the dominant medical group notices that it results in better service and proceeds to set it up. Let us pretend we are equal.

In the case described in this paper, nothing could have lessened the tremendous shock and loss experienced by the patient's family. The multitude of feelings experienced by the staff were extremely painful as well. We are all so alone. But what compounds the tragedy and many others like it is our inability at times like this to hold together, to share, to give comfort, to take comfort. To suggest that sex-role stereotyping and ranking are the sole contributors to this estrangement would be presumptuous; to ignore the factors in our system that so routinely assault our self-esteem and diminish our ability to care would be indefensible.

Implications and recommendations: The artificial separation of educational experiences for doctors and nurses plays a large part in maintaining the distance we see here. Doctors have long contributed to nursing education. Although doctors' lectures are no longer common in nursing education per se, hospital in-service programs for nurses still rely heavily on doctor as teacher of nurse and rarely if ever on nurse as teacher of doctor. Nurses have and do contribute a great deal to medical education, but always informally, usually in a game-playing manner, and certainly without recognition or reimbursement. "The Doctor Nurse Game" describes this unique teaching method whereby the nurse tells the doctor something in such a way that he is allowed to feel it was his idea in the first place (Stein, 1967).

Certainly, new and more equitable ways of educating people for human health care service need to be developed. We need to educate ourselves for teamwork, recognizing the unique expertise that different health-care team members contribute but also dealing with areas of overlapping in ways that promote self-esteem for all members. Medical and nursing schools should begin some dialogue to search for ways to break down existing barriers. Research needs to be done and published to substantiate the charge that sex-role stereotyping and ranking does in fact inhibit high-quality care for the sick and dying. Hospital administrators must begin to take some responsibility for promoting teamwork by not allowing the internal structure of the organization to continue to institutionalize ranking based on role stereotyping. In-service education departments should be encouraged to develop joint committees to design learning experiences to be shared by all caregivers. The problems are both complex and numerous.

They reflect attitudes pervasive in the entire society. Understanding the problem in its most human context, as it affects how we care for the dying person, can be a beginning step in recognition of the need for change toward more humane attitudes and practices.

REFERENCES

Krant, M. J. 1972. "The Organized Care of the Dying Patient." *Hospital Practice* (January):101–8.

Stein, L. I. 1967. "The Doctor Nurse Game." *Archives of General Psychiatry* 16 (June):669–703.

17

The Existential Meaning of Death

PETER KOESTENBAUM

The following analysis illustrates a specific application of the existential theory on the meaning of death in life (Koestenbaum, 1971). It is a response to a question raised by a public health nurse attending a seminar I directed.

QUESTION: I am a public health nurse. I work with dying children (leukemia, cancer), with their parents, and with dying oldsters. How can existential philosophy help me help my patients?

ANSWER: The first rule is for you to achieve authenticity in the area of death yourself. You must understand, first, the full *theoretical* spectrum of the existential philosophy of death and dying, and, second, you must have learned to fully integrate these intellectual insights into your *experience* and into your life. In other words, to help your patients, you yourself must be ready to die today. But there is more: You must also be able to die with dignity as if you were now a child; furthermore, you must also be capable of managing your life as the parent of a dying and then a dead child; and finally, you must also be able to die as an oldster, even in agony and loneliness. Once you are ready, you can help your patients.

If you have gone through the intellectual work of understanding and then through the emotional work of coming to terms with these issues, then the practical question of how to help your patients is relatively minor. Most of what is then needed for you, as an authentic person, is to make yourself available to your patients. Individuals who seek mere *techniques* for the management of the emotionally stricken may in reality wish to bypass any personal involvement with the personal commitment to the afflicted patient. However, it is precisely this ability to make a commitment to the patient that will help him. When the nurse seeks techniques, she is in effect asking to be transformed into a health machine that will "cure" philosophical or existential ills automatically, forgetting that love, devotion, and commitment are what heal philosophic ills such as inevitable death. The belief that a purely technological approach to inevitable death is even theoretically possible is evidence of total inauthenticity; it is proof of having completely misunderstood the nature of man.

The second rule is to understand the philosophical elements in the management of death. These make up the heart of an existential personality theory and can be summarized as follows:

An individual whose life is relatively uneventful will manage death with modest success if he adopts the first solution to what in existential philosophy is called "the paradox of self-transcendence," that is, conscious *repression* of philosophical themes. Many people go through life easily without ever seriously contemplating death. You, however, as a public health nurse, have made the contemplation of death your profession, the center of your life.

What does the knowledge of death do to the healthy individual? Only when that question is answered can we deal with the sick. In your case, the healthy ones are the *parents* of dying children. To them, the philosophical truth about death means the discovery of life's true values and life's true limits.

Confronted with death—any death whatever—a mouse's, a child's, a grandparent's, a stranger's, or his own—an individual immediately recognizes which values are important and which are not. Translated into the language of a nurse speaking to parents, this insight means she should focus not only on the values lost but also on the value remaining—and still to be created and to be achieved. For instance, there may be other children—if not, the parents might have or adopt additional children. The values of being a child and of being a parent remain. In fact, the death of a child immeasurably enhances the values of *all* children and of *all* parents. The death of a child sanctifies the values of childhood and parenthood. True, the love for the new children can never make up for the lost child. But new children are loved more intensely, warmly, and meaningfully, with a love nurtured on the soil of the dead child. And that nutriment makes all the difference because it sharply focuses the divine value of a human consciousness.

Furthermore, the dying of their child is limitation per se for the parents. Death is coming; that is a fact. No one and nothing can change that fact. And that fact is bad; it is the worst that can happen to them. It is the fate and nature of man to be condemned to these boundaries, these impenetrable barriers, these insurmountable walls. To be human is to be thus (unfairly) limited. And to be human is also to genuinely want to live with these boundaries; that is the difference between the infinity of God and the finitude of man. To *want* to be human is to want to be limited. And the ability to confront death is the proof of that want.

How can a public health nurse get these ideas across to the parents of a dying child? She can focus on the reality of the situation. She can emphasize that the child *will* die and call attention to this rather than ameliorate the fact that death is indeed a horrible tragedy and an unconscionable injustice, without redemption. She can help nature make clear to the parents that they, as human beings, are absolutely limited. We are all the prisoners of our humanity. She must avoid all statements that indicate there is hope for the child or that his death will not be so bad as was originally thought. The burial of the child is necessary—painful as it is for the family—to make clear to all the absolute finality of the act of death. That finality must be faced and confronted even before the death of the child.

The nurse might help by calling attention to *other* limits in their and others' lives. The parent himself may have lost a parent, or he may even have lost his own childhood in the war or the depression. He may have lost the opportunity for education or for the playing of a musical instrument. These are all irrecoverable limits—as was the marriage of his true childhood sweetheart to another person. Thus, to those who are well and to the survivors of the dead, a philosophical analysis of death enhances their seriousness about life by showing them man's true values and realistic limits.

But this approach is for the living, not for the dying, since these comments regarding the confrontation with our limits are for the healthy only. Death vitalizes only those who can reasonably expect to do some substantial and heady living. Those who are about to die must be treated far more gingerly and on different principles. Death has a different meaning for those who know they are about to die. In determining what approach to take, the crucial question the nurse must answer is "What is my patient's concept of death?"

Since no one living has died, the death of subjective consciousness is but a speculative belief. True, it is this belief that makes us human; however, children have not yet been taught this belief—oldsters know it by heart.

An old person must be given serious hope for the indestructibility of consciousness. That can be done through philosophical analysis (Koestenbaum, 1971, chs. 18, 19) or religious metaphor. The dying patient who has had time to prepare himself is peaceful and even joyous. He experiences the peace of one who knows that he is an indestructible consciousness that is not necessarily involved with the world. The dying person who is reconciled in this fashion has become, in effect, the saintly ascetic revered by all the world cultures in all the periods of history.

You would like to be able to tell your dying patients,

"Death is not the end," but you cannot in good conscience always say so. You, as a nurse dealing with the dying, hope that the notion of immortality—that is, the idea that consciousness is an Eternal Now and that time is outside the consciousness, an object to consciousness rather than an integral part of consciousness itself—can be supported philosophically. Can you accept that? Can you accept it theoretically? Practically and feelingly?

Here is a letter from a friend that, in the context of Alcoholics Anonymous, begs to substitute the philosophical idea of the indestructible consciousness for the religious belief in immortality:

Just some quick comments about the chapter in your book about "Phenomenology of Religion." As you know, because of my AA training I have come to depend a great deal upon a "Higher Power" to get sober and to stay sober in AA. For ten years this "Higher Power" has been represented by my "AA Group." I have not been able to accept the "God Concept" or the "Spiritual Thing" because of my disastrous 16 years of Catholic schooling. I am now ready to accept intellectually and emotionally your phenomenological concept of "my pure subjective consciousness" as my "Higher Power." However, I would like your personal comments to me about this—perhaps on the phone later this week, if possible.

The writer suffers from the death of God. He hopes the existential notion of pure consciousness can serve as a substitute. A concept alone cannot take the place of a living experience and vibrant reality. He needs a friend, one who cares and who loves, one who is permanently and fully available—a person who should have been but was not present in his childhood. He needs evidence of another consciousness connected to his consciousness. It is not enough for him to understand the principles of existential philosophy, he must also experience their meaning in the way he lives. Existential philosophy cannot be understood fully in one's study—any more than one can live fully there. Understanding means also action and, above all, relations with people, commitment to

people, and responses from people—interactions of conscious-
nesses.

The child, however, does not really know that he is dying.
He does sense the anxiety of his parents and thus fears something dreadful, even worse than death itself. His life must,
nevertheless, continue normally, unchanged, with hope, tenderness, and the full presence and availability of the consciousness of the parents.

When a child has hope, he possesses, in effect, an unadul-
terated sense of time. To be alive in the world means to have
become time. Time is always directed into the future. To experience time as a continuum that is rooted in the present
and uses the past to point to the future is the authentic experience of time. A dying child must retain the sense of authentic time—the future for him must always exist. It is the
privileged challenge of the parents and the nurse to create an
emotional and educational environment for the child in
which he can lead a future- and growth-oriented life, without
deceit. The child must now enjoy a humanistic education:
literature and the arts, philosophy and religion, and, above
all, the love and intimacy of other human beings.

Shakespeare expressed himself masterfully on death when
he wrote:

Cowards die many times before their deaths,
The valiant never taste of death but once.
Of all the wonders that I yet have heard,
It seems to me most strange that men should fear;
Seeing that death, a necessary end,
Will come when it will come. (*Julius Caesar,* Act II, Scene 2)

There are the basic points to remember:

To help others with death, you must first have come to
terms with your own death, intellectually and emotionally.

Specifically, you must have made your peace with these
four types of dying: (1) your death now; (2) your death if you
were now a child; (3) the death of your child now; and (4)
your death as an old and ailing person.

Techniques to help the dying are meaningless, since death

is a philosophical problem rather than a medical one. Remember, there is no cure for death!

To help the dying, you must understand the existential ideas on death. Many people repress the fact of death—knowledge of death helps us understand the true values of life; knowledge of death helps us understand the true limits of human existence.

The nurse must point out the increase in the remaining values and in obligations because of the finitude of man, made apparent by the death of a child.

The question of the eternity of consciousness should be raised with adults.

Children should live on without change in their life-styles; they must have hope and a sense of time that moves into the future.

REFERENCES

Koestenbaum, P. 1971. *The Vitality of Death, Essays in Existential Psychology and Philosophy.* Stamford: Connecticut Greenwood Press.

SEE ALSO

Koestenbaum, P. 1974. *Managing Anxiety: The Power Of Knowing Who You Are.* Englewood Cliffs: Prentice-Hall, Inc.

———— 1974. *Existential Sexuality: Choosing to Love.* Englewood Cliffs: Prentice-Hall, Inc.

———— 1976. Is There an Answer to Death? Englewood Cliffs: Prentice-Hall, Inc.

Education

PART THREE

18

〰〰〰〰〰〰〰〰〰〰〰〰〰〰〰〰

Teaching to Individual Differences

BEVERLY CAPACCIO FINEMAN

If one considers that life and death occur on a continuum, one's eventual nonbeing can be accepted by most individuals; death's finality is most likely projected far off into a nebulous future. Students, in their new careers in nursing, do not automatically become able or willing to deal with dying and death as reality simply because they have entered a profession that places death on a continuum with life.

If we agree with the hypothesis that the patient who is aware he is dying wishes to verbalize his feelings about the loss of his self, we must accept that the student nurse wishes to discuss her own new and growing awareness of death and dying as she meets these happenings on her daily rounds. To quote Kubler-Ross (1969, p. 31), "Death is always associated with impending death, a destructive nature of death, and it is that which evokes all the emotions." The way the nursing student handles her emotions relating to death is what most concerns the teacher. The student who avoids a dying patient by "forgetting" to carry out parts of her clinical assignment, and thus ensures a minimal need for her to enter the patient's room, is initiating a pattern of avoidance to deal with her feelings about those who are dying and the demands they might make of her.

The individual's response is determined by previous experiences with loss and death, by his methods of coping with pain, by cultural prescriptions available for handling the fact of death, and later by the structure of his professional identity (Schoenberg et al., 1970, p. 4).

Drawing on the individual differences of a student, as well as on the characteristics that students share in common, an astute teacher can stimulate them to contribute attitudes, feelings, and experiences related to loss and grief. Any one group of students will most likely represent a variety of cultures; and since each culture has its own stigmata concerning death, it has been the experience of this author that young students may need the "permission" of an authority (i.e., the teacher) to discuss attitudes, feelings, and experiences openly.

Diagnosis of the individual differences within a group of students is vital to the success of the teacher's plan. One must ask, "Who are the students, and what experience has each had with loss and grief?" Most individuals have probably had an experience with a dying person by the time they have reached college age. The rare individual who has not can be encouraged to air attitudes based on personal philosophy or garnered from readings, as well as from other vicarious experiences.

Teaching to individual differences in a group where attitudes will be explored is most successful if, in advance of the class, the objectives are written in terms of student behaviors, enabling students to be aware of what is expected of them and of any preparation to be done; if the style in which the class is to be conducted (e.g., discussion, role playing, seminar) is made clear; if students contribute willingly to the teacher's information about an experience with a dying person and certain personal data about themselves (age, marital status, cultural background); and if the student's willingness to discuss in a group her experiences with loss has been expressed. Such information will enable the teacher to develop a profile of each student and will allow her to draw on the differences and the similarities within the group.

It is important to select examples relevant to students' experiences and knowledge, to relate the examples to the principles or ideas being taught (de Tornyay, 1971, p. 24). Allowing students to present examples relevant to the concepts being taught and related to the objectives offers both student and teacher an opportunity to explore existing attitudes and new ideas.

The use of individual differences as a teaching strategy is excellent as a method of introducing students to loss and grief, for it draws on a wide range of past experiences in addition to the present difficulties the student is facing in dealing with these concepts. It is hoped that relating the real-life experiences of the students to each stage of the grieving (or dying) process will enable students to recognize grieving in patients. Most importantly, it is hoped that, by becoming aware of how patients handle loss, the student can conceptualize loss in a broader sense and use the cognitive skills gained to deal with her own needs and those of the patient.

The initial discussion of loss and grief was instituted in a discussion group consisting of seven students and one teacher. One student, a widow returning to college after raising her family, offered to describe the feelings of loss she had felt after her husband's sudden death from a myocardial infarction. Not only did her description aid her in emotional catharsis, but she was also able to describe succinctly and objectively her use of denial and subsequent isolation from her family.

I couldn't believe he was gone—it didn't seem possible. He was always so strong, only 46. For months after he died, I set a place for him at the table. When repairs were needed in the home, I would think, Jay will do it when he gets in. I found myself spending more time alone in order to think about Jay and our life together.

Her poignant response prompted others in the group to add examples of their uses of denial and isolation over the loss of a loved one—not necessarily by death—and of how defense mechanisms were used.

Most of the students were able to cite examples of anger. Primarily, the examples were those of patients who projected their feelings of rage and helplessness at the students who, in turn, were equally helpless in their ability to deal with what they saw as hopelessness and fearful of questions these patients might ask them about their illness. Students described examples of dealing with such patients by "asking for a change in assignment, never going into the patient's room, not 'seeing' the room light," and other avoidance techniques. It was necessary for the students to realize that anger and projection were safety valves for patients. Once the use of anger was explored by the students, nearly all of them could cite incidents in their own lives where loss had been the impetus for angry reactions. It was at this point in the discussion that the group began to understand that all loss involves some degree of grieving, and they could understand it within a conceptual framework.

Bargaining was more difficult for students to identify from their experiences. Bargaining meant a postponement, which included a prize for good behavior (Kubler-Ross, p. 83). Because most bargaining takes place between the patient and his deity, this form of defense is not always obvious to the observer. One of the students was able to contribute an excellent example of bargaining involving the loss of a loved one by separation.

I was eight when my parents separated. I stayed with Mother, and Daddy went to live in a hotel. Mother never really explained why Daddy had gone, just that he wasn't happy. I use to lie in bed at night and plead with God to send Daddy back. I promised I would always be cheerful, and he would be happy.

This student was also able to recollect her feelings of anger at God and at her mother when her father did not return home and, in fact, went to another city to live. She spent many months after that fantasizing that her father would send for her—she would always be cheerful—and she vacillated between bargaining and anger until she finally accepted that the situation was permanent. The teacher used this incident to point out that stages of grieving could overlap, and patients can actually progress and regress and progress from one stage to another.

It was then that the group predicted that depression would be a natural outcome of bargaining—when the bargaining is unsuccessful or the grieving person passes beyond that stage. The major problem in this part of the discussion was not how to recognize depression, though this can be difficult, but how to aid the patient who is in the depressive phase of grieving.

When the depression is a tool to prepare for the impending loss of all the love objects, to facilitate acceptance, then encouragement and reassurance are not as meaningful; that is "if [he] is allowed to express his sorrow, he will find a final acceptance much easier" (Kubler-Ross, p. 87).

It was difficult for the students to envision a situation wherein they could feel comfortable with a person as he expressed his unhappiness, mourning for his past and for his lost future. One student expressed her feelings as shyness and guilt at being made aware of another person's private feelings. Another student, who described herself as a "reserved type," had feelings of revulsion at being so close to sorrow. It was important for the group to describe and work out the feelings they had about allowing another to be sorrowful before the teacher could direct the activity toward nursing actions that could aid in the expression of sorrow. As one student put it, "The hardest thing in the world is to sit by while someone is crying over a loss or wrong and be expected to encourage the person to continue crying."

Acceptance, described as the "ideal" final stage, should not be mistaken for a happy stage. It is almost void of feelings. It is as if the pain is gone, the struggle is over, and there comes a time for the final rest before the long journey (Kubler-Ross, p. 113).

Emily, the widowed student, explained how she had finally completed mourning and accepted her loss:

I made the decision to return to college, not because I would need a livelihood in the future; nor was it something to fill in my time. I simply found myself ready to continue on, to start growing again, but in a way that was different. I'll never forget my life with Jay, but now I can plan a life without him.

The use of individual differences as a teaching strategy appeared to be successful in that the major objective—introducing the students to the concept of loss and the process of grieving—was met; examples relevant to students' experiences were used to relate examples to the actual concepts being taught. It was especially encouraging to note that students were very supportive of each other; knowing that only information volunteered to the teacher could be discussed in the group (in addition to what the student wished to add in the class), they were willing to contribute and face openly their attitudes and feelings.

REFERENCES

de Tornyay, R. 1971. *Strategies for Teaching Nursing.* New York: John Wiley and Sons.

Kubler-Ross, E. 1969. *On Death and Dying.* New York: Macmillan.
Schoenberg, B. et al., eds. 1970. *Loss and Grief: Psychological Management in Medical Practice.* New York: Columbia University Press.

19

Let The Teacher Beware!

JOSEPH R. PROULX

I propose to speak to the obvious because of the ever-increasing popularity of death education courses on college campuses and in professional schools across the country. In effect this article is intended as a road sign to warn faculty to slow down and to consider some of the implications of undertaking these courses. Although the desirability and necessity of having more programs on death education, particularly in schools that prepare health-care workers, are not being questioned, what is suggested is that courses on death and dying are sui generis.

In his novel *The Case Worker,* George Konrad (1974, p. 17) describes a past occupational experience:

I spent six months of my military service in an engineer squad, clearing mine fields. All around us the world was at peace, but we were at war. It wasn't just the money, the oranges, and the chocolate that appealed to us, or even the pride in belonging to a special unit. We were also attracted by what was virtually a game of chance. Every morning, though of course we took every precaution, we diced with death.

I am deeply indebted to Dr. Lisa Robinson (Associate Professor) and Mrs. Mary Watermann, R.N., M.S. (Instructor), both of the faculty of the University of Maryland School of Nursing. In personal interviews with them they graciously shared their thoughts, feelings, and words related to the preparation of this article.

Granted that this may be an overdramatized analogy, it is my intent to suggest that the occupation of teaching—and I refer here specifically to teaching courses on death and dying—has inherent dangers analogous to those of clearing a mine field. Of course, in working with explosives, the ultimate peril might lie in physical harm, whereas work with students in death education programs might involve psychological threats.

Courses dealing with death and dying broach societal taboos and personal hangups. The very nature of the subject matter is volatile, and hence, caution is urged in handling this topic.

One might hypothesize that the student of death vicariously experiences the same emotions, to a degree, as does the dying person himself, or as a significant other person who comes face to face with the news of the imminent death of a loved one (Leviton, 1972, p. 8).

Warning: defuse with care!

THE PROBLEM

Originally, this article was designed to address itself to the "inherent dangers" of a course in death and dying. I was intrigued by the apparent lack of any specific headings on this notion, despite the assistance of a computerized search of the literature. To be sure, caveats do appear. For example, "students still complained that more feelings were being evoked than could be dealt with. That, it seems to me, is one of the unavoidable hazards of teaching about death" (Anderson, 1972, p. 10). Also, "Whatever the approach, and whatever the focus of the session, it is very important to be aware of the emotional reactions that will be aroused among the students" (Simpson, 1973). However, the particular flavor of "danger" as a unique topic seemed to be missing. Interviews with two learned colleagues—both experienced death educators—helped to shed some light on this conundrum.

The respondents were asked the following question:

"What, if any, are the inherent dangers for students engaged in a death and dying course?" The replies are as follows:

I don't use that word [danger] much—it is not in my vocabulary. What we are talking about is challenging. It has to do with any kind of course in sensitivity. If you start bringing to the surface some stuff that has been lying there, that has been gnawing away at somebody . . . that had to be either consciously or subconsciously part of the motivation for taking the course.

I would say that there are no inherent dangers but for some students who tend to be depressed themselves or are having problems with their parents, these kids [sic] sometimes get into trouble.

Obviously, the danger symbol has become attenuated. In its place is an opportunity for increased awareness, self-growth, and an exploration of problem-solving potential. To illustrate these positive elements, one of my colleagues reported the following vignette.

One of the students was having problems with her mother. She had lost her grandmother early in the spring and her Mom had apparently had a very untoward reaction to the whole thing. And this student was able to talk about it in class and report that she was taking all the information from class home to her mother and the two of them were able to work out "their thing" during the spring semester.

By this time it had become increasingly clear to me that, though I might be in the right church, I was certainly not in the right pew. If the concept of "danger" was to persist, the focus must shift from the student to the teacher. The death educator is the person responsible and held accountable for the development of course content and process. The problem issue thus moved to: "What dangers are present for teachers of death and dying courses?"

THREATS TO THE TEACHER

"Teaching a course on death surfaces the split between the emotional and the cognitive in education in general" (Anderson, 1972, p. 12). If so, the death educator is laid open to both personal and professional hazards. In line with the former the teacher faces the same exposure as the student does. Leviton has summarized these threats as: (1) concern over the impending death or the past death of a loved one; (2) suicidal thinking, either as a continuous preoccupation or as a trenchant here-and-now possibility; and (3) thanatophobia— intense preoccupation with the thought of personal death (Leviton, p. 6). The teacher must live with his own finiteness as well as that of significant others.

Moreover, the teacher in a professional school is often looked upon as a role model, and this presents a peculiar situation for the instructor in death education. As one of my interviewees suggested,

The thing that makes a very effective caretaker for a dying patient versus someone else who is superficial is that the very effective person is the one who has transcended the need to deny his mortality. And these people I think are very rare. If the caretaker doesn't get over that hump then he can't really get involved with the patient to the extent that is necessary.

The death educator would seem to be particularly vulnerable to guilt stemming from possible deficiencies in both personal and professional domains. Three questions may be raised here. First, does the teacher present a healthy balance in his own personal and professional life? Second, is the teacher competent and comfortable in the role of death educator? Lastly, what about the rare—yet distinct—possibility of a student's suicide?

An integrated self-concept is necessary for the death educator, since this person must face his own feelings as well as bear the transient depression of the students. In addition, the hallmark of a death course is the intimacy established between teacher and learner. The exploration of death calls for sharing: teacher and students disclose themselves. A stable personality on the part of the teacher is necessary to but not sufficient for death education. The teacher must be viewed as a warm, caring human being; a nonmoralist; and an effective problem solver.

In the teacher role itself it is expected that the leader have a strong grasp of the subject matter plus a variety of alternatives for presenting this content. The selection of one or more modalities in evolving the course material should be based on the objectives of the curriculum as well as the individual needs of the students. It is also strongly urged that the death educator be fairly sophisticated about counseling and crisis intervention techniques if the need should arise to use these (Leviton, p. 2).

The threat of a student's suicide is best summed up as follows:

The instructor in Death Education needs to be prepared for the eventuality of a student's suicide. Not only will he have his own guilt feelings to work through but the news media and citizens' groups may blame the course material and the instructor, himself, for the death (Leviton, p. 6).

In more personal terms one of the nurse educators interviewed expressed her feelings about this awesome dilemma: "what I fear most is getting a student in the course who is in existential despair; one who has abandoned all hope. I don't know what I would do."

A salient point to be considered under the heading of professional dangers is the legal ramifications of the teacher's actions and those of his students. Again, this may be more clearly seen if we consider teaching a course to physicians and nurses as opposed to teaching the same course to a group of lay people. Ideas that may be discussed with impunity in the classroom may not be translated into action in the clinical setting without possible dire consequences. I refer here specifically to euthanasia, which is receiving widespread attention in medical ethics. In short it is one thing to discuss and even support the patient's "right-to-die" in the classroom. It becomes something entirely different if the student "pulls the plug" at the bedside while stating: "My teacher said . . ." Full awareness of the current legal constraints involved in such issues is an absolute necessity for the death educator. Then, too, the idea of confidentiality in the clinical setting must be understood by the instructor and stressed to the students. Indiscretions in naming patients, citing institutions, and reporting actions or inactions of health-care professionals must be guarded against.

PRECAUTIONARY MEASURES

The following suggestions are offered as guidelines to the death educator in general and the novice teacher in this area in particular. It is hoped that adherence to these somewhat simplistic and manifest dicta will make any course on death and dying less dangerous to the teacher and more profitable and enjoyable for the student.

First of all, the *teacher needs to be available.* Ample time should be given over to individual counseling and consultation for students. To facilitate this, the instructor should post regular office hours and adhere to them. It is also advisable for the instructor to give the students his home phone, so that he may be reached in case any problems arise during extracurricular hours.

The death educator should also have someone available to him. *Psychiatric supervision or guidance*—from colleagues within the school setting or therapists without—may be employed by the teacher for purposes of self-growth, and in times of crisis situations that might arise during the course. In this latter vein I refer to the sharing of particularly difficult problems posed by certain students or the alleviation of troublesome guilt that the instructor might be burdened with. In addition to professional support the teacher should have other authentic contacts and interests in his personal life from which positive "strokes" may be obtained when necessary.

The teacher's use of *language and humor* is crucial in providing a nonthreatening atmosphere in the classroom. Depending upon the background of the audience and the depth to which the subject matter is to be explored, the death educator should gradually introduce the language of death. It is not desirable to break down the student's defense mechanisms (specifically denial) too rapidly. The investigation of the subject matter requires a steady and articulate approach. In this context the use of humor may be viewed as a positive defense against anxiety that supports both student and teacher as they plumb the taboo. Humor should be used frequently at the appropriate times throughout the course; the teacher should bear in mind that its greatest efficacy comes in dealing with low to moderate levels of anxiety.

Some instructors use what I prefer to call *screening techniques* to assess the student's readiness or motivation in enrolling in a death and dying course. The two most common techniques used are the introductory statement and the Draw-A-Picture-of-Death exercise. The introductory statement is a brief personal report on why the student has elected to take the course. In sharing his personal motivation, the student begins to divulge himself to others. The instructor notes the degree of openness in the presentation, the student's comfort or discomfort in sharing with others, and any marked incongruencies between the speaker's words and expressions. In the latter artistic exercise, after drawing a picture, each student is asked to explain the creation to the class. This affords the instructor—and other students as well—yet another glimpse of the individual and his perception of death.

Many courses on death and dying require the students to submit weekly logs or diaries. These summaries contain a written report of each student's thoughts, feelings, and responses to any aspect of the course. The teacher uses these reports as guidelines to individual growth as well as a monitoring device to detect incipient emotional problems. Inherent in this requirement is the assumption that the death educator will carefully check each student's log regularly. Many times the student will be able to share information in this private manner that he is unwilling to share in a group context.

For professional students particularly, class size becomes important. Ideally, courses on death and dying should have a

216 JOSEPH R. PROULX

limited enrollment. A small class is conducive to individual student–teacher contact. The small group allows the instructor to get a more valid grasp of where each student is in terms of both course content and process. Certainly, for the teacher of such a proposed group an awareness of group dynamics is essential.

In an area where the subject matter itself is so threatening students must be given every opportunity to participate as freely as possible without the additional burden of academically induced anxiety. For this reason, the level of competition in the course needs to be reduced. For example, where freedom and openness are encouraged, it often becomes difficult for the instructor to evaluate a student's classroom participation. This is not to suggest that academic standards should be reduced. Rather, it is a warning to the instructor to search for methods (one that comes readily to mind is the Pass–Fail grading option) of student evaluation that allay rather than produce anxiety. As in any other educational offering, course requirements and the criteria for evaluation should be made explicit at the outset.

SUMMARY

At the very beginning the reader was cautioned that the content of this article might appear obvious. However, the cautionary notes contained herein bear review. For the death educator to be better prepared to fulfill his personal and professional responsibilities, he must be cognizant of the inherent dangers in teaching courses on death and dying. The teacher—particularly the apprentice—should be aware of these perils of possibilities before undertaking such a venture.

Specifically the question was asked: "What dangers are present for teachers of death and dying courses?" Although the general slant of the information contained herein is designed for professional school (medicine, nursing, etc.) educators, it is felt that the content is applicable for death educators everywhere. A brief discussion of some of the personal and professional risks involved in teaching death education courses was undertaken, and guidelines to mitigating these dangers were suggested.

REFERENCES

Anderson, 1972. "Learning and Teaching about Death and Dying." ERIC Document No. ED 075 728. Princeton, N.J.: Princeton Theological Seminary.

Konrad, G. 1974. *The Case Worker*. New York: Harcourt, Brace Jovanovich, Inc.

Leviton, D. 1972. "Education for Death, or Death Becomes Less a Stranger." ERIC Document No. ED 073 378. Rockville, Md.: National Institute of Mental Health, 1972.

Simpson, M. A. 1973. "Teaching about Death and Dying," *Nursing Times* 69 (April 5):442–43

20

Continuing Education in Aging and Long-Term Care

ELEANOR C. FRIEDENBERG

Only in recent years have health-care personnel really come to grips with the issues of death and dying. The orientation of educational programs and service practice of professionals dealing with care of the sick and injured was one of life-sustaining heroics in the emergency room and the operating room; valiant attempts on the medical–surgical units of hospitals and other health-care facilities to keep vital organs functioning with drugs and other artificial mechanisms such as heart-lung machines, tube feedings, and artificial kidneys; feelings of guilt and frustration when life-sustaining activities failed and the patient was pronounced dead. In fact, in many instances, the patient had ceased to live long before he was pronounced dead. One writer's chastisement of the medical profession (National Institute of Mental Health, 1971): is perhaps somewhat overstated but also valid:

When confronted with losing we do all kinds of things to prove we are trying to do good, do-gooders that we are. Surgical residents do radical neck dissections on octogenerians. We put feeding tubes in poor old bodies that should be allowed to die. Rehabilitation people break their backs to get old hemiplegics to take feeble steps for no purpose. We cannot admit to ourselves that death is a part of living.

Eric Hodgins, a former editor and author and a survivor of a serious stroke, believes

doctors too often treat the patient and ignore the person. . . . at my last bedside I want an individual who is understanding and compassionate . . . one who will never confuse the prolongation of my life with the prolongation of my death (Mannes, 1974).

Several issues are created for health care personnel as a factor of this orientation: at what point is the decision made that life-sustaining attempts are futile; who should participate in that decision; what can be done to permit an individual to participate in his own dying process in a manner that is comfortable and constructive for him; how can family or significant others participate in this process in a nonthreatening way; what is the role of personnel, especially nurses, who tend to have closest daily contact with patients and family, in providing support; and how are personnel prepared to perform this supportive role? This article is principally concerned with the last two issues, more specifically within the setting of the long-term health-care facility.

It is apparent that many professionals, especially physicians and nurses, have been concerned with issues of dying and death for some time. For a variety of reasons, however, only within recent years have they been dealt with in an open and objective fashion. Nursing curricula, until relatively recently, may have dealt with care of the body after death but rarely with how to provide total physical and emotional care of the dying person. There is almost a nonfocus on death in the experiences planned for students of nursing (Browning and Lewis, 1972). To have discussed how to help a person die would have seemed antithetical to good nursing education a decade ago. As one writer states:

We are at the same stage with dealing with death and terminal illness (now) as with talking about sex a generation ago (Moss, 1966).

The acknowledged pioneer in opening up discussion among health professionals about the many issues related to death and dying is Elisabeth Kubler-Ross. In her book *On Death and Dying* (1969) Dr. Kubler-Ross describes the resistance, at times hostility, that she encountered from personnel when she first began interviewing terminally ill patients, discussing with them their feelings about dying, their expectations of the staff's caring for them, and how the knowledge of their impending death affected family relationships. Dr. Kubler-Ross's experience was that the patients themselves were better able to handle the knowledge of terminal illness, in general, than their families or the persons caring for them were! Whereas the patient was ready, sometimes eager, to discuss the fact of his dying, health-care personnel tended to avoid such discussions—partly owing to unresolved anxiety regarding their own mortality, partly owing to not being able to accept their inability to cure, but mainly owing to plain ignorance about how best to cope with the situation—something their professional training had not prepared them to handle.

Dr. Kubler-Ross's work was conducted principally in an acute care hospital with patients in the young and middle-aged adult years. Whereas the principles she developed, awareness of the various stages of dying, and techniques for management of the dying patient are generally universal, there are factors that are somewhat unique to the long-term-care facility, with its predominantly geriatric population—a population usually suffering from more than one chronic or disabling illness.

An image of nursing homes or long-term-care facilities, commonly held especially by the aged, is that it is only a place to *go and die* (Garvin and Berger, 1968). Tremendous psychic energy on the part of administrators and staff and especially of public relations personnel in the long-term-care field is expended in denying this image. In fact, the nursing home *is* a place to *go and die* for the majority of persons admitted. Approximately 90 percent of all discharges from nursing homes in a recent Michigan study were by death (Gottesman, 1973). Thirty percent of all new admissions expired within three months. With these kinds of statistics, it is no wonder that nursing home personnel are sensitive about their public image. Dr. Alvin Goldfarb, a psychiatrist with extensive experience in long-term-care facilities, notes that:

the high rate of death in the first few months is undoubtedly due to their moribund/pre-terminal condition on admission. It seems doubtful that the provision of extra services greatly prolongs life in the very ill, although it may add immeasurably to comfort (Busse and Pfeiffer, 1969).

It is certainly not to be denied that a major emphasis of long-term care should be rehabilitative, or at least restorative, care. Data suggest that, in any type of institution, with adequate shelter, food, and general medical care, the life span of the severely impaired and disabled aged persons is related to their physical condition, or viability, upon admission. Conversely, the relatively well may live somewhat longer in facilities that have programs and services that contribute to pleasure and the maintenance of dignity. That maintenance of dignity must continue through the life-terminating as well as the life-sustaining process. As recently as December 6, 1973, the *Washington Post* reported that the American Medical Association for the first time took an official position on the "death with dignity" issue.

Consequently, it seems incumbent on personnel in long-term-care facilities to be prepared to serve two key functions, which at first glance might appear to be antithetical but are actually two interrelated parts to a continuum of care. The first is, of course, the generally accepted role of providing skilled care aimed at restoring or maintaining the patients-residents' maximal functioning. Furthermore, since the average length of stay in the long-term-care facility is two years (Gottesman, 1973), it is imperative that personnel strive to maintain as homelike an environment as possible. Any place a person resides in for two or more years must be considered home. The staff of the facility becomes a kind of surrogate family, whether or not the resident has a real family, and assumes many of the functions that a family would normally assume.

The other key function of the long-term-care facility, and by far the more difficult one, is providing an environment in which terminally ill residents can die in peace, with dignity, aided by persons who are understanding, empathetic, and supportive of their needs, and those of their families and fellow residents. This is acknowledged to be a tall order and a function for which the majority of long-term-care personnel have not been prepared. As our society in general becomes more free about discussing dying and death, this function will be less difficult for long-term-care personnel. Conversely, these personnel are in a key position to facilitate this freedom. This can be accomplished, for those already in the field, only by a process of continuing education sanctioned by administrators and conducted in such a way as to permit open expression of anxiety, fear, and uncertainty on the part of personnel. This step is necessary before it becomes possible to discuss the constructive ways in which personnel can be supportive to others. There must also be developed an acceptance of the value of the role of the long-term-care facility as a place to die with dignity when that point in life has been reached.

In dealing with the dying patient, staff must be aware of when he is ready and able to talk, and structure the situation in such a way that the patient can know when staff members are ready to listen. Being able to pick up cues of readiness is a skill that can be learned. In all instances, but particularly in those, not infrequent in long-term-care facilities, when the dying person is unconscious, the staff must learn to be particularly sensitive to the family's needs. Families of residents are frequently punished by staff, who tend to feel the family has dumped or abandoned the elderly relative to the care of the facility because they do not wish to care for him. In fact, in all too many instances, families have waited too late to make an institutional placement, because of the stigma, when an earlier placement would have been in everyone's best interest.

(Busse and Pfeiffer, 1969). We have a vicious cycle going here that must be broken—another issue.

Particularly with the old person who may have had a slow, lingering process of death, personnel are faced with a combination of family grief, hostility, and ambivalence toward the dying one (Poe, 1972). Personnel must be able to assist the family in accepting and verbalizing their real feelings—for instance, it is permissible to feel burdened, drained by the dying process. They are not to be blamed for wishing it were all over—staff members frequently feel the same way. When the dying is finished, it is all right to cry openly, and for the personnel who have at times been a surrogate family it is all right for them also to cry. Fellow residents must be allowed to share in the dying process as they are able or want to—no more closing of doors and surreptitious removing of the dead person, pretending death did not happen.

The only educational format for accomplishing these goals that seems feasible to this writer is one based on the adult-education principle of shared learning. That is, based on the assumption that adult learners have a lifetime of skills, knowledge, and attitudes and bring these with them to the learning situation. Where necessary skills and knowledge are lacking in the group, this is sought from the outside in a way that is relevant to the group's needs. Where an individual's needs are not consistent with movement toward a goal, defined by the learner group, these are examined by the total group for both cause and validity. If necessary, individual work is then done with a given learner. Particularly in a subject area as emotionally laden as death and dying, anxieties and misconceptions on the part of the learner group must be dealt with first, before the staff can be expected to deal in a constructive and helpful way with the dying person and his family.

The learning process may start with the personal experiences staff members have had with the deaths of friends, relatives, and acquaintances. The staff should be encouraged to explore how they felt, how their own needs were or were not met at the time. This exploration helps personnel identify with the feelings of the family and friends of the dying patient as well as gain some insight into their own unresolved conflicts about death, which may be interfering with their effectiveness as supporting persons. Continuing-education programs might also start with explorations of the literature on death, both fiction and nonfiction, to provide learners with a common starting base. No long-term-care facility can be said to provide total care until its personnel are prepared to accept and function in the role of assisting with the *dying* process with the same skill and understanding they have with the *living* process.

The American Nurses Association has noted that ability to deal with issues surrounding death is an integral part of geriatric nursing. In the recently developed Standards of Geriatric Nursing Practice, Standard II reads, in part:

THE NURSE SEEKS TO RESOLVE HER CONFLICTING ATTITUDES REGARDING AGING, DEATH AND DEPENDENCY SO THAT SHE CAN ASSIST OLDER PERSONS AND THEIR RELATIVES TO MAINTAIN LIFE WITH DIGNITY AND COMFORT UNTIL DEATH ENSUES

Rationale: If the nurse does not recognize and seek to resolve conflicts regarding aging, death and dependency, functioning can be impaired and personal satisfaction not be achieved from her work. These conflicts are resolved to enable the nurse to enlarge her capacity to express empathy and compassion. Dying and death are common emotional and stressful experiences. Preparation for death is an imminent developmental task of old age. The older person is more frequently exposed to dying and death. The nurse needs to assist older persons who are experiencing dying, death and bereavement in order that they may express their feelings, thoughts and rituals.

In summary, it is my position that an ongoing process of continuing education is essential for the implementation of this as well as the other geriatric nursing practice standards. This is particularly true for personnel in long-term-care facilities, where the large majority of patient discharges are by death. The continuing-education process can assist in legitimizing the role of the long-term-care facility as a place to die with dignity. Furthermore, it is only through continuing education that personnel can develop the knowledge and skills needed to participate in total professional care of the patient during the period of dying.

REFERENCES

Browning, M. H., and E. P. Lewis, eds. 1972. *The Dying Patient: A Nursing Perspective.* New York: American Journal of Nursing Company.

Busse, E. W., and E. Pfeiffer, eds. 1969. *Behavior and Adaptation in Late Life.* Boston: Little, Brown and Company.

Garvin, R. M. and R. E. Burger. 1968. *Where They Go to Die: The Tragedy of America's Aged.* New York: Delacorte Press.

Gottesman, L. E. 1973. Unpublished paper presented at a "Workshop on Coordination of Long-Term Care Services," U.S. Department of Health, Education, and Welfare (December 4).

Kubler-Ross, E. 1969. *On Death and Dying.* New York: Macmillan.

Mannes, M. 1974. *Last Rights.* New York: Morrow.

Moss, B. B. 1966. *Caring for the Aged.* New York: Doubleday.

National Institute of Mental Health. 1971. "It Can't Be Home." DHEW Publication HSM 71–9050. Washington, D.C.: U.S. Government Printing Office.

Poe, W. D. 1972. "Marantology, A Needed Specialty." *The New England Journal of Medicine* 286 (January):102–3.

ADDITIONAL BIBLIOGRAPHY

de Beauvoir, S. 1972. *The Coming of Age.* New York: G.P. Putnam's Sons.

Schwab, Sister M. L. 1968. "The Nurses' Role in Assisting Families of Dying Geriatric Patients to Manage Grief and Guilt." *ANA Clinical Sessions.* New York: Appleton–Century–Crofts.

Stone, V. 1969. "Nursing of Older People." In *Behavior and Adaptation in Late Life,* eds. E. Busse and E. Pfeiffer. Boston: Little, Brown and Company.

Walker, M. 1973. "The Last Hour before Death." *American Journal of Nursing* 73 (September): 1592–93.

Death Influence in Clinical Practice:

A Course Outline for the Nursing School Curriculum

JEANNE QUINT BENOLIEL

This course was conducted by the author at the School of Nursing, University of Washington, Seattle, Washington. It is presented here as a model for similar courses to be included in the curricula of other institutions.

THE EDITORS

COURSE DESCRIPTION

Analysis and study of social, cultural, and psychological conditions that influence human death in modern society. Research findings, selected readings, and direct experience provide direction for examination of philosophical, theoretical, and pragmatic issues underlying choices and decisions in clinical practice.
Prerequisite: Graduate standing and consent of instructor. (Enrollment limited to 16 students.)

COURSE OBJECTIVES

1. Become informed about the complex interrelationships of death practices in human societies to cultural norms, social structure, individual and collective belief systems, and historical forces.

2. Broaden perceptions of the psychosocial and cultural meanings of death and the differential effects of socialization on attitudes, beliefs, and practices through selected readings, group discussions, and direct experience in talking with other people about death.

3. Become sensitive to similarities and differences in individual and family attitudes toward and behavioral responses to death and

the conditions that influence these attitudes and behaviors through examination of research findings and reports of clinical studies.

4. Study and analyze similarities and differences in orientations toward death held by individuals and social groups whose work involves them in human death.

5. Compare and contrast the psychosocial consequences of expected and unexpected death for individuals, families, institutions, and the helping occupations.

6. Compare and contrast selected theoretical and conceptual orientations toward grief, mourning, and bereavement behaviors and explore the philosophical and pragmatic implications for clinical practice.

7. Identify and study the conflicts and pressures imposed by work that requires decisions of a life–death nature, the conditions that influence decisions to be made, and the effects of technological and social changes on choices available to practitioners in the health sciences.

8. Examine various moral, ethical, legal, and professional norms and codes of conduct pertaining to issues of life and death and explore the philosophical, practical, and problematic aspects of applying abstract principles to concrete social problems.

COURSE EXPECTATIONS

1. Discussion in seminar is based on readings, instructor and student knowledge from prior contacts with death, and experience derived from laboratory assignments.

2. Weekly assignments (4–6 hours) provide for direct experience in talking with people about death or in analyzing social situations concerned with death or dying. Both individual and group assignments are included.

3. Reading need not be limited to course requirements, and a lengthy list of references is available.

4. Two papers are expected.

    a. A formal paper deriving from the objectives of the course and the student's particular set of interests, and

    b. A written statement of philosophy underlying clinical practice as a professional service to people. The latter paper is not used for purposes of grading but to assist the student in formalizing his ideas about the many complex issues involved.

5. Opportunity is provided for individual and group evaluation of the content and methods used in the course.

TOPIC OUTLINE OF CONTENT

  I. Social Values and Death in Human Society
    A. Norms and codes of conduct as a reflection of cultural values—comparison of death practices in selected primitive societies used for illustration
    B. Analysis of death and social structure in modern, urban societies
    C. Emergence of thanatology as a field of investigation
  II. Occupations That Deal with Death in Modern Society
    A. Types of occupations concerned with death
    B. Specialization and division of labor in the provision of pre-death care (care for the dying)
  III. Institutional Death: Its Forms and Effects
    A. Types of institutions in which death takes place
    B. Differences in institutional death and dying
      1. Time
      2. Work orientations
      3. Death expectations
    C. Research reports bearing on death in institutions
  IV. Meaning of Death for the Family
    A. Family structure and the social consequences of death
    B. Grief and bereavement—a cross-cultural consideration of its meaning and manifestations
    C. The process of grieving—stages, critical junctures, and effect of interactions with other people, especially those who hold significant positions
  V. Life versus Death—An Occupational Dilemma for Physicians
    A. Changing context of medical practice
    B. Expectations, choices, and decisions faced by physicians in different areas of specialization
    C. Ethical, moral, and legal issues associated with changes brought by medical technology and with public and professional pressures
    D. Investigations and research concerned with the meaning of death to physicians

VI.   Recovery Care versus Comfort Care—Nurses' Perspectives and Problems
   A.   Types of contexts where nurses encounter death
   B.   Problematic aspects of work involving death
   C.   Reports of research bearing on the meaning of death to nurses
VII. Dying as Personal Experience
   A.   Perspectives on the meaning of dying drawn from psychoanalytic and psychiatric literature, personal descriptions, and fictional accounts, and interpretations by psychologists, sociologists, and writers in other fields
   B.   Circumstances that influence the meaning of dying
   C.   Modes of coping with forthcoming death
VIII. Effect of Dying on Social Interaction
   A.   Social isolation as a consequence of being defined as dying
   B.   Psychosocial stages of dying and the grieving process
   C.   Effects of bereavement on physical and mental health
   D.   Grief—its normal and abnormal manifestations
   E.   Appropriate and inappropriate interventions in clinical practice—a comparison of recommended approaches
IX.   Socialization for Care of the Dying
   A.   High priority attached to life-saving activity and the consequences for curricula in the health science fields
   B.   Present status of teaching about death and dying in schools of medicine and nursing and social work
   C.   Psychosocial care for the dying as a form of work— theoretical, philosophical, practical, and problematic issues
   D.   Problematic aspects of bringing about changes in priorities
X.   Unresolved Questions and Major Issues
   A.   Ethical, moral, legal, and philosophic issues pertaining to human choices and actions where life and death of another human being are at stake, for example, organ transplants, abortion, use of life-maintaining equipment, genetic manipulations

B.   The individual's right to live and die in his own way versus society's rules and regulations for the common good

C.   Guidelines for clinical practice—the relationship of personal philosophy to professional choice

GUIDELINES FOR ASSIGNMENTS

1.   Group Assignment—to investigate the social management of human death in the community-at-large. Some areas of concern:

a.   Characteristics of persons who die—analysis of vital statistics in newspapers and other resources as appear pertinent

b.   Ways of dying that "make news"—analysis of reports presented via TV, newspapers, and other modes of communication to the public

c.   Facilities where death occurs—analysis of local community to get a general picture of settings where death occurs with some frequency, for example, numbers and types of hospitals, nursing and convalescent homes, living areas for the elderly, and other types of custodial institutions

d.   Facilities for handling death—analysis of community to determine numbers and locations of funeral homes, cemeteries, crematories, and other organizations concerned with death.

You are to divide into four groups—each group determining its division of labor and approach to the task. Be prepared to discuss in class.

2.   *Group Assignment*—to investigate occupational groups whose work requires them to deal with death (excluded are health workers). Some categories of "death work":

a.   Work that requires killing (armed forces, police, law enforcement agencies, executioners, etc.)

b.   Emergency and death prevention (ambulance drivers, policemen and firemen, emergency room staffs, suicide prevention workers, etc.)

c.   Post-death work, both legal and social (morticians, funeral directors, coroner, morgue attendant, cemetery and mausoleum workers, worker in crematoria, etc.)

d.   Counseling relative to death (clergy, psychiatrists, lawyers, psychologists, mental health workers, etc.).

You are to divide into four groups—each group making its own decision on how to proceed with the task as follows. Find out: (1) how people are prepared for work that involves death; (2) what kinds of tasks must be done by them; (3) how they feel about their work; and (4) what aspects they find especially difficult. Discussion in class.

3. *Group Assignment*—care for the dying is an occupational task for many persons employed in hospitals and other types of institutions. The organization of work by the staff depends on *how much* and *what kind* of death they encounter on a regular basis. You are being asked to collect some sociological data about dying and its management in several different settings: emergency room, cancer ward, pediatric ward, general medical ward, general surgical ward, a nursing home or convalescent hospital, or others. For this assignment you are to work in pairs.

For purposes of analysis you will be interested in such factors as: (1) frequency of death; (2) type of death most common to setting; (3) characteristics of the clientele who are served (socioeconomic status, ethnic, and personal backgrounds, etc.); (4) number and types of occupational groups providing services; and (5) spatial handling of death. For discussion, you are asked to consider these questions:

    a.   How open or visible is death or dying, and how is visibility managed?

    b.   Where are dying patients located spatially and/or temporally in relation to other patients, family, regular staff, and outsiders?

    c.   What kind of division of labor is practiced with respect to death care—who does what tasks?

    d.   What are major problems encountered by staff—as they see them, as you see them?

4. *Individual Assignment*—to broaden your understanding of the effects of death on families, you are asked to talk with five people who are different in terms of such variables as age, sex, occupation, marital status, race, religion, ethnic background, and other elements. You are to include strangers and persons you know.

From each person you are trying to learn:

    a.   whether he has experienced death in his immediate or extended family (how many, who, when, etc.)

b.   whether any one death was especially meaningful

c.   whether he and the family went through a period of active mourning, including any special rituals or activities

Preparatory for discussion in class, consider:

a.   what you have learned about death as a crisis event in the family

b.   what you have learned about grief and mourning and other aspects of adaptation to death by families and individuals

5.   *Individual Assignment*—you are asked to talk with five physicians about the problems that the dying patient poses for them. To obtain different perspectives, you are asked to select doctors who are different in terms of such characteristics as age, stage of medical practice, field of specialization, types of hospital used for practice, etc. In talking with each, you are trying to learn:

a.   what he sees as the most difficult problem for the physician in handling death

b.   in his own experience, what death stands out in his mind, and why

c.   what he sees as the nurses' most difficult problem in providing care for the dying patient

6.   *Individual Assignment*—You are to learn something about the continuing life experience of a person living with a life-threatening disease (either in the hospital or at home). The assignment requires that you be in contact with this person for some period of time— over several weeks. To understand his perspective you will need to spend time with him, allowing him ample time to talk about what is important to him. Try to arrange times so that you can chat together without interruption. You are trying to understand:

a.   what he is concerned about at this point in time

b.   what he knows about his condition and his future

c.   how he views his relationship with his family

d.   how he views the institutions providing his care, and the staff of that institution

7.   *Guidelines for Statement of Philosophy*

Before doing this assignment, you are expected to have read in preparation for the discussion dealing with unresolved problems and major issues relative to human death.

After giving the matter some serious thought, you are asked to put in writing your philosophy about (nursing) practice as a professional service to people. In making this statement, you are asked to consider how your philosophical position is influenced by these two forces: (1) the individual's right to live and die in his own way and (2) society's mandate to set and enforce rules and regulations for the common good (collective man).

Then describe how you plan to implement this philosophy in practice in the future (using the particular position that you intend to occupy) and what barriers you expect to encounter in providing the kind of service that you believe your clients (whether patients or students) deserve. The barriers are likely to come from several sources: within you, from other occupational groups or individuals, and the social structure of the institution within which you function.

Finally, what *specific steps* can you take to improve the services you presently offer to your clients—as compared with what you have done in the past? What *risks* must you take to make such a change? (Those who plan to offer secondary services rather than direct services to patients and families, for example, teachers and supervisors who direct and guide other individuals more directly engaged in providing direct care, will want to consider how you might function with these persons to provide them with assistance in coping with work that involves death.)

RECOMMENDED TEXTS

Kubler-Ross, E. 1969. *On Death and Dying.* Macmillan.
Quint, J. 1967. *The Nurse and the Dying Patient.* Macmillan.
Pearson, L. 1969. *Death and Dying: Current Issues in the Treatment of Dying Persons.* Cleveland: Case Western Reserve University Press.

USEFUL RESOURCES

Vernick, J. 1970. *Selected Bibliography on Death and Dying.* Washington, D.C.: National Institutes of Health, U.S. Government Printing Office.
Fulton, R. 1973. *A Bibliography on Death, Grief and Bereavement* (1845–1973). University of Minnesota: Center for Death Education and Research.
Patient Care 4 (May 31, 1970), issue devoted to "The Paradox of Death and the 'Omnipotent' Family Doctor."

JOURNALS: *Omega; Archives of the Foundation of Thanatology; Journal of Thanatology*

REQUESTED AND RECOMMENDED READINGS

TOPIC: *Social Values and Death in Human Society*

* Blauner, R. 1966. "Death and Social Structure." *Psychiatry* 29 (November): 378–94. (Also in *Middle Age and Aging,* ed. Neugarten. Chicago: University of Chicago Press).
* Volkart, E. 1965. "Bereavement and Mental Health." In *Death and Identity,* ed. R. Fulton. New York: John Wiley and Son. (Also in *Explorations in Social Psychiatry,* 1957, ed. A. H. Leighton, et al. New York: Basic Books).
* Mandelbaum, D. 1959 "Social Uses of Funeral Rites." In *Death and Identity,* ed. R. Fulton. New York: John Wiley and Sons; also, Feifel. H. 1959. *The Meaning of Death.* New York: McGraw-Hill.
Choron, J. 1963. *Death and Western Thought.* New York: Collier Books.
Choron, J. 1964. *Modern Man and Mortality.* New York: Macmillan.
Lester, D. 1970. "Religious Behavior and the Fear of Death." *Omega* 1 (August): 181–88.
Lifton, R. 1964. "On Death and Death Symbolism: The Hiroshima Disaster." *Psychiatry* 27: 191–210.
——— 1969. *Death in Life.* New York: Vintage Books.
Mathison, J. 1970. "A Cross-Cultural View of Widowhood." *Omega* 1 (August): 201–18.
Mitford, J. 1963. *The American Way of Death.* New York: Simon and Schuster.
Moore, J. 1970. "The Death Culture of Mexico and Mexican–Americans," *Omega* 1 (November): 271–91.
Robins, L. 1968. "Negro Homicide Victims—Who Will They Be?" *Trans-action,* 3 (June): 15–19.
Rossi, A. 1966. "Abortion Laws and Their Victims." *Trans-action,* 3 (September–October): 7–12.
Shneidman, E. 1969. "Prologue: Fifty-Eight Years." In *On the Nature of Suicide,* ed. E. Shneidman. San Francisco: Jossey-Bass.

* Indicates reference is requested reading before discussion in class.

Craven, M. 1973. *I Heard the Owl Call My Name.* New York: Doubleday.

TOPIC: *Occupations That Deal with Death in Modern Society*

* Quint, J. *The Nurse and the Dying Patient,* chs. 1 and 2.
* Kubler-Ross, E. *On Death and Dying.* Chapters 1 and 2.
* Fulton, R. 1965. "Sacred and Secular." In *Death and Identity,* ed. R. Fulton. New York: John Wiley and Sons.
* Jackson, E. 1959. "Grief and Religion." In *The Meaning of Death,* ed. H. Feifel. New York: McGraw-Hill.
Bittner, E. 1967. "Police Discretion in Emergency Apprehension of Mentally Ill Persons." *Social Problems* 14 (Winter): 278–92.
Bowers, M. K. et al., eds. 1964. *Counseling and Dying,* chapters 3, pp. 52–73. New York: Nelson.
Brim, O. et al. 1970. *The Dying Patient,* part 1, "Social Context of Dying," pp. 5–64. New York: Russell Sage Foundation.
Creighton, H. 1957. *Laws Every Nurse Should Know,* chapters 9 and 10, pp. 104–27. Philadelphia: Saunders.
Kastenbaum, R. and R. Aisenberg. 1972. *The Psychology of Death.* New York: Springer.
Raether, H. 1971. "The Place of the Funeral: The Role of the Funeral Director in Contemporary America." *Omega* 2 (August): 136–49.

TOPIC: *Institutional Death—Its Forms and Effects*

* Glaser, R. and A. Strauss. 1967. *Awareness of Dying,* parts I and II, pp. 3–115. Chicago: Aldine.
* ———— 1968. *Time for Dying,* chapters 3–7, pp. 30–147. Chicago: Aldine.
* Spitzer, S. and J. Folta. 1964. "Death in the Hospital—a Problem for Study." *Nursing Forum* 6, no. 4: 85–92.
McGinity, M. and B. Stotsky. 1967. "The Patient in the Nursing Home." *Nursing Forum* 6, no. 4: 85–92.
Roth, J. 1966. "The Public Hospital: Refuge for Damaged Humans." *Trans-action* 3 (July–August): 25–29.
Sudnow, D. 1970. "Dead on Arrival." In *Where Medicine Fails,* ed. A. Strauss, pp. 111–29. Chicago: Trans-Action Books.
———— 1967. *Passing On.* Englewood Cliffs, New Jersey: Prentice-Hall.

TOPIC: *Death and the Family*

* Stub, H. 1966. "Family Structure and the Social Consequences of Death." In *A Sociological Framework for Patient Care,* eds. J. Folta and E. Deck, pp. 191–200. New York: John Wiley and Sons.

* Kalish, R. 1969. "Effects of Death upon the Family." In *Death and Dying,* ed. L. Pearson, pp. 79–107. Cleveland: Case Western Reserve University Press.

* Kubler-Ross, E. *On Death and Dying,* Chapter 9.

* Engel, G. 1964. "Grief and Grieving." *American Journal of Nursing* 64 (September): 93–98.

Agee, J. 1957 *A Death in the Family.* New York: Avon.

Anderson, R. 1970. *I Never Sang for My Father.* New York: Signet Books.

Binger, C. et al. 1969. "Childhood Leukemia: Emotional Impact on Patient and Family." *New England Journal of Medicine* 280 (February 20): 414–18.

Fulton, R., ed. *Death and Identity,* Part III, "Grief and Mourning."

Gorer, G. 1967. *Death, Grief and Mourning.* Garden City, New York: Doubleday.

Gunther, J. 1949. *Death Be Not Proud.* New York: Harper and Company. (Paperback, Pyramid Books, 1960).

Hamovitch, M. 1964. *The Parent and the Fatally Ill Child.* Los Angeles: Delmar Publishing.

Hinton, J. 1967. *Dying.* Baltimore: Pelican Books.

Kutscher, A. H., ed. 1969. *Death and Bereavement.* Springfield, Illinois: Charles C Thomas, Inc.

Levinson, P. 1972. "On Sudden Death." *Psychiatry* 35 (May):160–73.

Meyerowitz, J. and H. B. Kaplan. 1967. "Familial Responses to Stress: The Case of Cystic Fibrosis." *Social Sciences and Medicine* 1:249–66.

Segal, E. 1970. *Love Story.* New York: Harper and Row.

Weisman, A. D. 1973. "Coping with Untimely Death." *Psychiatry* 36 (November):366–78.

TOPIC: *Life vs. Death: An Occupational Dilemma* (The Physician's Perspective)

* Glaser and Strauss, *Awareness of Dying,* Chapter 11, pp. 177–203.

* Ayd, F. 1962. "The Hopeless Case." *Journal of the American Medical Association* 181 (September 29):1099–1102.

* Lasagna, L., "Prognosis of Death" and "Physicians' Behavior toward the Dying Patient," In *Dying Patient,* ed. Brim, pp. 67–101.

* Vernon, G. 1970. *Sociology of Death,* pp. 298–314. New York: Ronald Press.

Davis, F. 1960 "Uncertainty in Medical Prognosis, Clinical and Functional." *American Journal of Sociology* 66 (July):41–47, reprinted in *Medical Care,* eds. Scott and Volkart, pp. 311–21. New York: John Wiley and Company.

Moore, F. 1965. *Give and Take,* chapters 9, 10, 11, pp. 149–96. New York: Doubleday–Anchor.

Scheff, T. 1972. "Decision Rules and Types of Error and Their Consequences in Medical Diagnosis." In *Medical Men and Their Work,* eds. Freidson and Lorber, pp. 309–23. Chicago: Aldine.

Tarnower, W. 1969. "The Dying Patient: Psychological Needs of the Patient, His Family and the Physician." *Nebraska State Medical Journal,* January, pp. 6–10.

Verwoerdt, A. 1966. *Communication with the Fatally Ill.* Springfield, Illinois: Charles C Thomas, Inc., especially Chapters 1–4, pp. 30–52.

Wasserman, N. 1967. "Problematic Aspects of the Phenomenon of Death." *World Medical Journal* 14 (September–October):146–49.

Artiss, K. L. and A. S. Levine. 1973. "Doctor–Patient Relation in Severe Illness." *New England Journal of Medicine* 288 (June 7):1210–14.

Crane, D. 1973. "Physicians' Attitudes toward the Treatment of Critically Ill Patients." *BioScience* 23 (August):471–74.

Cassell, E. J. 1973. "Permission to Die." *BioScience* 23 (August):475–77.

TOPIC: *Recovery Care vs. Comfort Care: Nurses' Problems*

* Glaser and Strauss, *Awareness of Dying,* chapters 12, pp. 204–25.
* Quint, *The Nurse and the Dying Patient,* chapters 5 and 6.
* Moss, F. and B. Meyer. 1966. "Effects of Nursing Interaction on Pain Relief in Patients." *Nursing Research* 15 (Fall):303–6.
* Vreeland, R. and G. Ellis. 1969. "Stresses on the Nurse in an Intensive Care Unit." *Journal of the American Medical Association* 208 (April 14):332–34.

* Quint, J. 1967. "The Dying Patient: A Difficult Nursing Problem." *Nursing Clinics of North America* 2 (December):763–73.
Davidson, R. 1966. "To Give Care in Terminal Illness." *American Journal of Nursing* 66 (January):74–75.
Geis, D. 1965. "Mothers' Perceptions of Care Given Their Dying Children." *American Journal of Nursing* 65 (February):105–7.
Hay, D. and D. Oken. 1972. "The Psychological Stress of Intensive Care Unit Nursing." *Psychosomatic Medicine* 34 (March–April):109–18.
Holsclaw, P. 1965. "Nursing in High Emotional Risk Areas." *Nursing Forum* 4, no. 4:36–45.
Jaeger, D. and L. Simmons. 1970. *The Aged Ill,* pp. 170–228. New York: Appleton-Century Crofts.
Nichols, E. 1972. "Jeannette: No Hope for Cure." *Nursing Forum* 11, no. 1:97–104.
Quint, J. 1967. "When Patients Die: Some Nursing Problems." *Canadian Nurse* 63 (December):33–36.
Regan, W. 1965. "The Legal Side of Confidential Information." *RN* (June): reprinted, 1967, in *Nursing Fundamentals,* ed. Meyers, pp. 69–73. Dubuque: Brown.
Vernick, J. and J. Lunceford. 1967. "Milieu Design for Adolescents with Leukemia." *American Journal of Nursing* (March): pp. 559–61.

Topic: *Dying as a Personal Experience*

* Kubler-Ross, E. *On Death and Dying,* chapters 3–7.
* Bard, M. 1966. "Price of Survival for Cancer Victims." *Transaction* 3 (March–April):10–14; reprinted in *Where Medicine Fails,* ed. A. Strauss. Chicago: Aldine.
* Butler, R. 1963. "The Life Review: An Interpretation of Reminiscence in the Aged." Psychiatry 26 (February); reprinted in *Middle Age and Aging,* ed. B. Neugarten. 1968. Chicago: University of Chicago Press.
* Quint, *The Nurse and Dying Patient,* chapter 7.
Bowers, M. K. et al. *Counseling the Dying,* chapter 2.
Browne, I. and T. Hackett. 1967. "Emotional Reactions to the Threat of Impending Death: A Study of Patients on the Monitor Cardiac Pacemaker." *Irish Journal of Medical Science* 6 (April):177–87.
de Beauvoir, S. 1966 *A Very Easy Death.* New York: Putnam.

Dovenmuehle, R. 1965. "Affective Response to Life-Threatening Disease." In *Death and Dying: Attitudes of Patient and Doctor, Symposium No. 11*, pp. 607–14. New York: Group for Advancement of Psychiatry.

Drugg, R. and D. Kornfield. 1967. "Survivors of Cardiac Arrest." *Journal of the American Medical Association* 201 (July 31):291–96.

Feder. S. 1965. "Attitudes of Patients with Advanced Cancer." In *Death and Dying: Attitudes of Patient and Doctor, Symposium No. 11*, pp. 614–22. New York: Group for Advancement of Psychiatry.

Grollman, E., ed. 1967. *Explaining Death to Children*. Boston: Beacon Press.

Hugos, R. 1972. "Living with Leukemia." *American Journal of Nursing* 72 (December):2185–88.

Kastenbaum, R. "Time and Death in Adolescence." In *Meaning of Death*, ed. H. Feifel, pp. 99–113.

Kimball, C. 1971. "Death and Dying: A Chronological Discussion." *Journal of Thanatology* 1 (January–February):42–52.

McCullers, C. 1962. *Clock without Hands*. Boston: Houghton-Mifflin (Paperback, New York: Bantam Books).

Noyes, R. 1972. "The Experience of Dying." *Psychiatry* 35 (May):174–84.

Quint, J. 1964. "Mastectomy: Symbol of Cure or Warning Sign?" *GP* 29 (March):119–24; reprinted in *A Sociological Framework for Patient Care*, eds. Folta and Deck.

Schoenberg, B. et al., eds. 1970. *Loss and Grief: Psychological Management in Medical Practice*, pp. 51–115; pp. 119–217; pp. 221–309. New York: Columbia University Press.

Solzhenitsyn, A. 1969. *The Cancer Ward*. New York: Bantam Books.

Weisman, A. D. and T. Hackett. 1961. "Predilection to Death." *Psychosomatic Medicine* 33:232–56; reprinted in *Death and Identity*, ed. R. Fulton.

TOPIC: *Effect of Dying on Human Relationships*

* Quint, *The Nurse and the Dying Patient*, chapter 4.
* Kubler-Ross, *On Death and Dying*, chapters 10 and 11.
* Quint, J. 1965. "Institutionalized Practices of Information Control." *Psychiatry* 28 (May):119–32.
* Crate, M. 1965. "Nursing Functions in Adaptation to Chronic Illness." *American Journal of Nursing* 65 (October):72–76.

Arteberry, J. 1967. "Distance and the Dying Patient." In *Current Concepts in Clinical Nursing*, eds. Bergerson et al., pp. 128–36. St. Louis: Mosby.

Benoliel, J. 1970. Talking to Patients about Death." *Nursing Forum* 9, no. 3:254–68.

Dudley, E. et al. 1969. "Long-Term Adjustment, Prognosis and Death in Irreversible Diffuse Obstructive Pulmonary Syndromes." *Psychosomatic Medicine* 4 (July–August):310–25.

Folta, J. 1965. "Perception of Death." *Nursing Research* 14 (Summer):232–35.

Friedman, S. 1963. "Behavioral Observations on Parents Anticipating the Death of a Child." *Pediatrics* 32 (October), Part I:610–25.

Heusinkveld, K. B. 1972. "Cues to Communication with the Terminal Cancer Patient." *Nursing Forum* 11, no. 1:105–13.

Knowles, L. 1962. "How Our Behavior Affects Patient Care." *Canadian Nurse* 58 (January):30–33.

Lowenberg, J. 1970. "Coping Behaviors of Fatally Ill Adolescents and Their Parents." *Nursing Forum* 9, no. 3:269–87.

Parkes, C. M. 1970. "The First Year of Bereavement," *Psychiatry* 33 (November): 444–67.

Quint, J. 1969. "The Threat of Death: Some Consequences for Patients and Nurses." *Nursing Forum* 8, no. 3, pp. 286–300.

Ryser, C. et al. 1971. "Problems with Change: The Vicissitudes of a Pilot Comprehensive Cancer Care Program." *Journal of Thanatology* 1 (May–June):145–55.

Saunders, C. "The Moment of Truth." In *Death and Dying*, ed. L. Pearson, pp. 49–78.

Sobel, E. 1969. "Personalization on the Coronary Care Unit." *American Journal of Nursing* 69 (July):1439–42.

Weismen, A. D. 1970. "Misgivings and Misconceptions in the Psychiatric Care of Terminal Patients." *Psychiatry* 33 (February):67–81.

TOPIC: *Unresolved Problems and Major Issues*

* Kubler-Ross, *On Death and Dying*, chapter 12.
* Quint, *The Nurse and the Dying Patient*, chapters 3 and 8.
* Clemence, Sister Madeleine. 1966. "Existentialism: A Philosophy of Commitment." *American Journal of Nursing* 66 (March):500–5.

* Savard, R. 1970. "Serving Investigator, Patient, and Community in Research Studies." In *New Dimensions in Legal and Ethical Concepts for Human Research,* Annals of New York Academy of Sciences, 169 (January 21):429–34.

* Koestenbaum, P. 1971. "The Vitality of Death." Omega 2 (November):253–71.

* Brim, O. et al., eds. *The Dying Patient,* pp. 211–302. See also, R. Glaser, "Innovations and Heroic Acts in Prolonging Lives, pp. 102–28.

Augenstein, L. 1969. *Come, Let Us Play God.* New York: Harper and Row.

Benoliel, J. 1971. "Assessments of Loss and Grief." *Journal of Thanatology* 1 (May–June):182–94.

Bowers, M. et al. *Counseling the Dying,* chapters 5–8.

Camus, A. 1959. *The Myth of Sisyphus and Other Essays,* pp. 88–91. New York: Vintage Books.

Camus, A. 1960. *Resistance, Rebellion and Death.* New York: Modern Library Series, Random House.

Fletcher, J. 1960. "The Patient's Right to Die." Harpers 221 (October):139–43.

Kass, L. 1971. "The New Biology: What Price Relieving Man's Estate." *Science* 174 (November 18):779–88.

Koop, C. 1968. "What I Tell a Dying Child's Parents." *Readers Digest* (February):141–45.

Kron, S. 1968. "Euthanasia: A Physician's View," and J. Leeman, "Euthanasia: Man's Right to Die." *Journal of Religion and Health* 7 (October):333–49.

Powers, T. 1971. "Learning to Die." *Harpers* 242 (June):72–80.

TOPIC: *Unresolved Problems and Major Issues* (continued)

Quint, J., A. Strauss, and B. Glaser. 1967. "Improving Nursing Care of the Dying." *Nursing Forum* 6, no. 4:368–78.

Simmons, R. and J. Fulton. 1971. "Ethical Issues in Kidney Transplantation." *Omega* 2 (August):179–90.

Schoenberg, B. et al., eds. 1972. *Psychosocial Aspects of Terminal Care.* New York: Columbia University Press.

Thaler, G. 1966. "Grief and Depression," and G. Ujhely, "Grief and Depression: Implications for Preventive and Therapeutic Nursing Care." *Nursing Forum* 5, no. 2:8–35.

Verwoerdt, A. *Communication with the Fatally Ill,* chapters 9 and 10.

Bok, S. 1973. "Euthanasia and the Care of the Dying," *BioScience* 23 (August): 461–70.

Meyers, D. W. 1973. "The Legal Aspects of Medical Euthanasia." *BioScience* 23 (August): 467–70.

The following articles from L. S. Bermosk and R. J. Corsini, eds. 1973. *Critical Incidents in Nursing.* Philadelphia: Saunders:

"Helping the Patient to Die," pp. 54–65.

"The Doctor Lets the Patient Die," pp. 127–33.

"Dignity in Dying," pp. 160–70.

"A Last Request," pp. 179–86.

"Induced Abortion," pp. 302–12.

"Caught in the Middle," pp. 313–24.

"A Conspiracy of Silence," pp. 325–33.

INDEX

Compiled By

LUCIA A. BOVE

CONTRIBUTORS

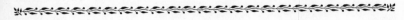

Nina T. Argondizzo, R.N., M.S., Assistant Dean, Cornell University-New York Hospital School of Nursing, New York, New York

Jeanne Quint Benoliel, R.N., D.N. Sc., Professor, Community Health Care Systems Department, University of Washington, Seattle, Washington

Lucia Bove, Publications Associate, The Foundation of Thanatology, New York, New York

Kenneth A. Chandler, Ph.D., Professor, Department of Psychology, Vassar College, Poughkeepsie, New York

A. Barbara Coyne, R.N., Associate Professor of Nursing, Duquesne University, Pittsburgh, Pennsylvania

Ann M. Earle, R.N., Ed.D., Associate Professor of Nursing, Department of Nursing of the Faculty of Medicine, College of Physicians and Surgeons, Columbia University, New York, New York

James S. Eaton, Jr., M.D., Chief, Psychiatry Education Branch, National Institute of Mental Health, Rockville, Maryland

Joseph F. Fennelly, M.D., Department of Internal Medicine, Morristown Memorial Hospital, Morristown, New Jersey

Beverly Capaccio Fineman, R.N., Assistant Professor, Department of Nursing of the Faculty of Medicine, College of Physicians and Surgeons, Columbia Universiey, New York, New York

Eleanor C. Friedenberg, M.S., R.N., Chief, Provider Improvement Branch, Division of Long-Term Care, United States Public Health Service, Department of Health, Education and Welfare, Rockville, Maryland

Nancy Proctor Greenleaf, R.N., M.S., Psychiatric Nursing, Boston University; Clinical Faculty, Boston State College, Department of Nursing, Boston, Massachusetts

Eileen Jacobi, Ed.D., R.N., Executive Director, American Nurses' Association, Kansas City, Missouri

Peter Koestenbaum, Ph.D., Professor of Philosophy, San Jose State University, San Jose, California

Liberty Kovacs, M.S., R.N., Mental Health Nurse Consultant and Assistant Clinical Professor, University of California at Davis, School of Medicine; Division of Mental Health, Sacramento Medical Center, Sacramento, California

Austin H. Kutscher, D.D.S., President, The Foundation of Thanatology, New York, New York

Lillian G. Kutscher, Publications Editor, The Foundation of Thanatology, New York, New York

Joan Liaschenko, Department of Radiation Therapy, Hahnemann Hospital and Medical Center, Philadelphia, Pennsylvania

June S. Lowenberg, R.N., M.N., Nurse Educator and Consultant (Private Practice); formerly, Lecturer, University of California School of Nursing, San Francisco, California

W. A. L. Lyall, M.D., Staff Psychiatrist, Clarke Institute of Psychiatry, Toronto; Associate Professor, Department of Psychiatry, University of Toronto

Joseph R. Proulx, Ed.D., Associate Professor, School of Nursing, University of Maryland, Baltimore, Maryland

Joy Rogers, Mental Health Consultant, Clarke Institute of Psychiatry, Toronto

John E. Schowalter, M.D., Director of Training and Professor of Clinical Pediatrics, and Psychiatry, Yale University Child Study Center, New Haven, Connecticut

Pauline M. Seitz, C.N.M., M.S.N., Nurse-Midwife; Associate Clinical Specialist, The New York Hospital-Cornell Medical Center, New York, New York

Yvonne Singletary, M.S., R.N., Psychiatric Clinical Nurse Specialist, Harlem Hospital Center, New York, New York

Richard J. Torpie, M.D., Department of Radiation Therapy, St. Luke's Hospital, Bethlehem, Pennsylvania

M. L. S. Vachon, R.N., Mental Health Consultant, Clarke Institute of Psychiatry, Toronto; Lecturer, Department of Psychiatry, University of Toronto

Lucy Warren, R.N., Assistant Professor of Clinical Nursing, Department of Nursing of the Faculty of Medicine, College of Physicians and Surgeons, Columbia University, New York, New York

Shirley L. Williams, R.N., M.N., Clinical Specialist, Chemotherapy Oncology, Veterans Administration Hospital, Minneapolis, Minnesota